ALSO BY ANNE BOYER

A Handbook of Disappointed Fate

Garments Against Women

The Romance of Happy Workers

THE UNDYING

THE UNDYING

__ PAIN,
_ VULNERABILITY,
_ MORTALITY,
_ MEDICINE,
__ ART,
_ TIME,
_ DREAMS,
_ DATA,
__ EXHAUSTION,
_ CANCER,
_ AND
_ CARE

ANNE BOYER

__
_
_
__
_
_
_

FARRAR, STRAUS AND GIROUX   NEW YORK

Farrar, Straus and Giroux
120 Broadway, New York 10271

Library of Congress Cataloging-in-Publication Data
Names: Boyer, Anne, 1973– author.
Title: The undying : pain, vulnerability, mortality, medicine, art, time,
    dreams, data, exhaustion, cancer, and care / Anne Boyer.
Description: First edition. | New York : Farrar, Straus and Giroux, 2019. |
    Includes bibliographical references.
Identifiers: LCCN 2019000373 | ISBN 9780374279349 (hardcover)
Subjects: LCSH: Boyer, Anne, 1973– —Health. | Breast—Cancer—
    Patients—United States—Biography. | Women authors, American—
    Biography. | Women artists—United States—Biography. |
    Cancer—Psychological aspects. | Mortality—Psychological
    aspects. | Literature—Psychology.
Classification: LCC RC280.B8 B645 2019 | DDC 616.99/4490092 [B]—
    dc23
LC record available at https://lccn.loc.gov/2019000373

Designed by Abby Kagan

Our books may be purchased in bulk for promotional, educational, or
business use. Please contact your local bookseller or the Macmillan
Corporate and Premium Sales Department at 1-800-221-7945, extension
5442, or by e-mail at MacmillanSpecialMarkets@macmillan.com.

www.fsgbooks.com
www.twitter.com/fsgbooks • www.facebook.com/fsgbooks

10 9 8 7 6 5 4 3 2 1

Not even if I had ten tongues and ten mouths.

—*The Iliad*

CONTENTS

PROLOGUE 1

THE INCUBANTS 11

BIRTH OF THE PAVILION 45

THE SICKBED 89

HOW THE ORACLE HELD 137

THE HOAX 163

IN THE TEMPLE OF GIULIETTA MASINA'S TEARS 203

WASTED LIFE 243

DEATHWATCH 259

EPILOGUE / and what it was that saved me 281

NOTES 293

BIBLIOGRAPHY 303

ACKNOWLEDGMENTS 307

PROLOGUE

In 1972, Susan Sontag was planning a work to be called "On Women Dying" or "Deaths of Women" or "How Women Die." In her journal under the heading "material," she wrote a list of eleven deaths, including the death of Virginia Woolf, the death of Marie Curie, the death of Jeanne d'Arc, the death of Rosa Luxemburg, and the death of Alice James.[1] Alice James died of breast cancer in 1892 at the age of forty-two. In her own journal, James describes her breast tumor as "this unholy granite substance in my breast."[2] Sontag quotes this later in *Illness as Metaphor*, the book that she wrote after undergoing treatment for her own breast cancer, diagnosed in 1974 when she was forty-one.[3]

Illness as Metaphor is cancer as nothing personal. Sontag does not write "I" and "cancer" in the same sentence. Rachel Carson is diagnosed with breast cancer in 1960, at the age of fifty-three, while in the process of writing *Silent Spring*, among the most important books in the cultural history of cancer. Carson does not speak publicly of the cancer from which she dies in 1964.[4] Sontag's journal entries during cancer treatment stand out for how few there are and how little they say. The little they do say illustrates breast cancer's cost to thinking, mostly as a result of chemotherapy treatments that can have severe and long-lasting cognitive effects. In February 1976, while undergoing chemotherapy, Sontag writes, "I need a mental gym." The next entry is months later, in June 1976: "when I can write letters, then . . ."[5]

In Jacqueline Susann's 1966 novel *Valley of the Dolls*, a character named Jennifer, afraid of mastectomy, dies by intentional overdose after her breast cancer diagnosis.[6] "All my life," Jennifer says, "the word cancer meant death, terror, something so horrible I'd cringe. And now I have it. And the funny part is, I'm not the least bit frightened of the cancer itself—even if it turns out to be a death sentence. It's just what it'll do to my life." The feminist writer Charlotte Perkins Gilman, diagnosed with breast cancer in 1932, kills herself, too: "I have preferred chloroform to cancer."[7] Jacqueline Susann, diagnosed at forty-four, dies of breast cancer in 1974, the year Sontag is diagnosed.

In 1978, the poet Audre Lorde is also diagnosed with breast cancer at the age of forty-four. Unlike Sontag, Lorde uses the words "I" and "cancer" together, and does this famously in *The Cancer Journals*, which includes an account of her diagnosis and treatment and a call to arms: "I don't want this to be a record of grieving only. I don't want this to be a record only of tears." For Lorde, the crisis of breast cancer meant "the warrior's painstaking examination of yet another weapon."[8] Lorde dies of breast cancer in 1992.

Like Lorde, the British novelist Fanny Burney, who discovers her breast cancer in 1810, writes a first-person account of her mastectomy.[9] Her breast is removed without anesthetic. She is conscious for the mastectomy's duration:

> . . . not for days, not for Weeks, but for Months I could not speak of this terrible business without nearly again going through it! I could not think of it with impunity! I was sick, I was disordered by a single question—even now, 9 months after it is over, I have a head ache from going on with the account! & this miserable account . . .

"Write aphoristically," Sontag notes in her journal when contemplating how to write about cancer in *Illness as Metaphor*.[10] Breast cancer exists uneasily with the "I" that might "speak of this terrible business" and give "this miserable account." This "I" is sometimes annihilated by cancer, but sometimes preemptively annihilated by the person it represents, either by suicide or by an authorial stubbornness that does not permit "I" and "cancer" to be joined in one unit of thought:

> "[Redacted] is diagnosed with breast cancer in 2014, at
> the age of forty-one."
> or
> "I am diagnosed with [redacted] in 2014, at the age of
> forty-one."

The novelist Kathy Acker is diagnosed with breast cancer in 1996, at the age of forty-nine. "I am going to tell
this story as I know it," begins "The Gift of Disease," an
uncharacteristically straightforward account she wrote
about cancer for *The Guardian*: "Even now, it is strange
to me. I have no idea why I am telling it. I have never been
sentimental. Perhaps just to say that it happened." Acker
doesn't know why she would tell the story and yet she
does: "In April of last year, I was diagnosed as having
breast cancer."[11] Acker dies of it in 1997, within eighteen
months of being diagnosed.

Although breast cancer can happen to anyone with breast
tissue, women bear the substantial weight of its calamities. These calamities come to women with breast cancer
by way of early death, painful death, disabling treatment,
disabling late effects of treatments, loss of partners,
income, and capacity, but the calamities also come via
the social morass of the disease—its class politics, gendered delimitations, and racialized distribution of death,
its rotating scheme of confused instructions and brutal
mystifications.

If few diseases are as calamitous to women in effects as breast cancer, there are even fewer as voluminous in their agonies. These agonies are not only about the disease itself, but about what is written about it, or not written about it, or whether or not to write about it, or how. Breast cancer is a disease that presents itself as a disordering question of form.

The answer to that question of form is often competing redactions and these redactions' interpretations and corrections. For Lorde, a black lesbian feminist poet, the redaction is cancer's, and the silence around the disease is an entrance to politics: "My work is to inhabit the silences with which I have lived and fill them with myself until they have the sounds of brightest day and loudest thunder."[12] For Sontag, an upper-class white cultural critic, the redaction is of the personal. As she wrote in a note under prospective titles for what would become *Illness as Metaphor*: "To think only of oneself is to think of death."[13]

A fourth title Sontag proposed for her never-to-be-written piece was "Women and Death." She claims, "Women don't die for each other. There is no 'sororal' death." But I think Sontag was wrong. A sororal death would not be women dying for each other: it is death in an alienated parallel. A sororal death would be women dying of being women. The queer theorist Eve Kosofsky Sedgwick, diagnosed with breast cancer in 1991, at the age of forty-one, wrote about breast cancer culture's startling, sometimes brutal impositions of gender. Sedgwick, at her diagnosis, wrote that she thought, "Shit, now I guess I really must be a woman."[14] As S. Lochlann Jain writes in a chapter called "Cancer Butch" in the book *Malignant*, "one charming little diagnosis threatens to suck you under, into the archetypal death doled out by the feminine body."[15] Sedgwick died of breast cancer in 2009.

Women might not, as Sontag claimed, die for each other, but their deaths by breast cancer are not without sacrifice. At least in the age of "awareness," that lucrative, pink-ribbon-wrapped alternative to "cure," what we are told must be given up for the common good is not so much one's life as one's life story. The silence around breast cancer that Lorde once wrote into is now the din of breast cancer's extraordinary production of language. In our time, the challenge is not to speak into the silence, but to learn to form a resistance to the often obliterating noise. Sontag's and Carson's reluctance to link themselves to the disease has now become replaced with an obligation, for those women who have it, to always do so.

Though I might claim, as Acker did, to not be sentimental, this sentence joins myself and my breast cancer together in—if not a sentimental story—at least an ideological one:

"I was diagnosed with breast cancer in 2014, at the age of forty-one."

Breast cancer's formal problem, then, is also political. An ideological story is always a story that I don't know why I would tell but still do. That sentence with its "I" and its "breast cancer" enters into an "awareness" that becomes a dangerous ubiquity. As Jain describes it, silence is no longer the greatest obstacle to finding a cure for breast cancer: "cancer's everywhereness drops into a sludge of nowhereness."[16]

Only one class of people who have had breast cancer are regularly admitted to the pinkwashed landscape of awareness: those who have survived it. To those victors go the narrative spoils. To tell the story of one's own breast cancer is supposed to be to tell a story of "surviving" via neoliberal self-management—the narrative is of the atomized individual done right, self-examined and mammogramed, of disease cured with compliance, 5K runs, organic green smoothies, and positive thought. As Ellen Leopold points out in her history of breast cancer, *A Darker Ribbon*, the rise of neoliberalism in the 1990s brings a change in breast cancer's narrative conventions: "the external world is taken as a given, a backdrop against which the personal drama is played out."[17]

To write only of oneself is not to write *only* of death, but under these conditions, to write more specifically of a type of death or a deathlike state to which no politics, no collective action, no broader history might be admitted. Breast cancer's industrial etiology, medicine's misogynist and racist histories and practices, capitalism's incredible machine of profit, and the unequal distribution by class of the suffering and death of breast cancer are omitted from breast cancer's now-common literary form. To write only of oneself may be to write of death, but to write of death is to write of everyone. As Lorde wrote, "I carry tattooed upon my heart a list of names of women who did not survive, and there is always a space for one more, my own."[18]

In 1974, the year she was diagnosed with breast cancer, Sontag writes in her journal: "My way of thinking has up to now been both too abstract and too concrete. Too abstract: death. Too concrete: me." She admits, then, what she calls a middle term: "both abstract and concrete." The term—positioned between oneself and one's death, the abstract and concrete—is "women." "And thereby," Sontag added, "a whole new universe of death rose before my eyes."[19]

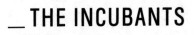

_ THE INCUBANTS

1.

When the technician leaves the room, I turn my head toward the screen to interpret any neoplasms, the webs of nerves, the small lit fonts in which my pathology and/or future or future end might be written. The first tumor I ever saw was a darkness on that screen, round with a long craggy finger jutting from it. I took a photo of it from my exam table with an iPhone. That tumor was my own.

I learned I was sick at the cusp of clinic and sensation. I wore the same green tank top, cutoffs, and sandals that I wore every summer—then surprise, then grim persuasive professional rhetoric filling up the climate control, that serious woman in a gray suit emphatic about the doom, then personal panic, clinical refinements, astonished Gchats with my friends. An investigator enters my life dressed up as an entire social institution, says they are launching an investigation into sensations a person (me) hasn't yet had to feel, but will.

To take a set of objects and actions from one system and reclassify these as elements in another system is like fortune-telling. To a fortune-teller, birds flying north spell out tomorrow's happiness and tea leaves tell a story about two lovers and the third who will ruin them. After that, the flight of the birds has been freed from the meaning "migration," and when it has become a tale about the future end of the lovers, the tea is no longer anything we want to drink.

To take a thing or set of things from one system and re-classify these as elements in another also resembles diagnosis, which takes information from our bodies and rearranges what came from inside of us into a system imposed from far away. My lump was once in the system of me, but the moment the radiologist gave it a BI-RADS 5 score, it became a tumor forever at home in the system of oncology.[1] Like the birds that have been liberated from the content of their flying and like the liberated tea, a diagnosed person is liberated from what she once thought of as herself.

To be declared with certainty *ill* while feeling with certainty *fine* is to fall on the hardness of language without being given even an hour of soft uncertainty in which to steady oneself with preemptive worry, aka *now you don't have a solution to a problem, now you have a specific name for a life breaking in two.* Illness that never bothered to announce itself to the senses radiates in screen life, as light is sound and is information encrypted, unencrypted, circulated, analyzed, rated, studied, and sold. In the servers, our health degrades or improves. Once we were sick in our bodies. Now we are sick in a body of light.

Welcome to the detectors with names made of letters: MRI, CT, PET. Earmuffs on, gown on, gown removed, arms up, arms down, breathe in, breathe out, blood drawn, dye injected, wand in, wand on, moving or being moved—radiology turns a person made of feelings and flesh into a patient made of light and shadows. There are quiet technicians, loud clatters, warmed blankets, cinematic beeps.

An image in a clinic isn't: it is *imaging*. We who become patients through the waves and stopped waves of sono-grams, of light tricks and exposures, of brilliant injectable dyes, are by the power vested in me by having-a-body's universal law now to be called *the imagelings*. "Come in with a full bladder," the technicians say on the phone to the imagelings, wanting to look into our interesting inte-riors. The sonogram that can find a new life in a person's womb can also find an embryonic death there.

We fall ill, and our illness falls under the hard hand of science, falls onto slides under confident microscopes, falls into pretty lies, falls into pity and public relations, falls into new pages open on the browser and new books on the shelf. Then there is this body (my body) that has no feel for uncertainty, a life that breaks open under the alien terminology of oncology, then into the rift of that language, falls.

There are people who feel bad in their bodies and do nothing about it, and there are people who feel bad in their bodies and submit their symptoms to search engines and stop there. Then there are people who can afford to circulate what hurts between professionals who will offer them competing diagnostic bids. This group of people follow a set of symptoms toward a promise, ask for tests, question answers, travel long distances to visit specialists who might be able to recognize what's wrong.

If symptoms are circulated long enough, a set of discomforts might be allowed the mercy of a name: a disease, a syndrome, a sensitivity, a search term. Sometimes that is cure enough—as if to appellate is to make okay. Sometimes to give a person a word to call their suffering is the only treatment for it.

In a world where so many people feel so bad, there's a common unmarked and indefinite state of feeling ill that provides, at least, membership in a community of the unspecified. Discomfort in need of diagnosis forms a feeling-scape of curious pains and corporeal eruptions, all untamed by the category *disease*. The kind of illness that has no name is the kind that is held in suspense or held in common or shuffled into the adjacency of psychiatry.

A body in mysterious discomfort exposes itself to medicine hoping to meet a vocabulary with which to speak of suffering in return. If that suffering does not meet sufficient language, those who endure that suffering must come together to invent it. The sick but undiagnosed have developed a literature of unnamed illness, a poetry of it, too, and a narrative of their search for answers. They finesse diets in response to what medicine fails, assay lifestyle restrictions, and in the mix of refined ingestion and corrective protections and rotating professional inspections, health or ill health wanders from the bounds of medicine, resists both disease and cure.

Cancer's custom, on the other hand, is to rarely show up unannounced. Cancer comes in a wave of experts and expert technologies. It arrives via surveillance and professional declaration. Our senses tell us almost nothing about our illness, but the doctors ask us to believe that what we cannot see or feel might kill us, and so we do.

"They tell me," said an old man to me in the chemotherapy infusion room, "I have cancer, but," he whispered, "I have my doubts."

But we knew that something was wrong, that the world was wrong (catastrophically), that we were wrong (catastrophically), that something (anything) was catastrophically wrong everywhere.

We were sick in a gloss of total health, and totally healthy in a sickening world.

We were lonely, but unable to form the bonds necessary to end our loneliness.

We were overworked, but intoxicated by our own working.

I thought I had become sick (in a manner), that I was unwell (in the spirit), that I was collapsing in a fit of Faustianism in a devil's bargain world.

2.

Aelius Aristides, a Greek orator born during the reign of Nero, tried to heal his illness by sleeping in the sacred territory of the god Asclepius and obeying the instructions of dreams. Aristides, who was twenty-six when he fell ill, lived for years among the incubants in Asclepius's temple in Pergamum. There, the sick waited for divine prescriptions from Asclepius to appear as they slept, and when the sick woke, they followed them. Now we sleep in the precincts of gods we have forgotten, statistics an ulterior mysticism.

Our century is excellent at the production of nightmares and terrible at the interpretation of dreams. Asleep, I break into the Whole Foods near Oakland's Lake Merritt with an oncologist who praised the way I dress. Or Madonna is in two of my classes with her breasts exposed. I am in a village for a purpose, and I have too much equipment to haul, and there are famous people, but I can't remember who. I get in a debate about all the world and about all the heavens, and a man I am debating sends me a message: "I am trying to figure out from what center you come."

A newly diagnosed person with access to the Internet is information's incubant. Data visits like a minor god. Awake, we pass the day staring into the screen's abyss, feeling the constriction of the quantitative, trying to learn to breathe through the bar graphs, head full of sample sizes and survival curves, eyes dimming, body reverent to math.

The newly installed chemo port hurts. The nurses tell me chemo ports hurt more the younger you are. They tell me that everything about cancer hurts more. I resist bathing and grooming, stop moving freely. I don't think about the other parts of my body, what they can still do, because the one part that hurts causes the others to fade from awareness. Someone sends me a link to a baking soda cancer cure. A former student emails to ask if I have heard about juicing.

Aelius Aristides writes his book of dreams sent to him from the god Asclepius, *Hieroi Logoi*, in the early 170s, years after his initial illness and during the anxious years of the reign of Marcus Aurelius.[2] Asclepius was said to be the son of a mortal woman and Apollo and raised by a centaur who instructed him in the art of medicine. In one version of his story, Asclepius was such an effective medical practitioner that Hades had him killed out of fear of an empty underworld. Not only is *Hieroi Logoi* a record of prescriptive dreams, but it is also an autobiographical account of what it is like to have a body in a specific time and place. Sacred dreamers took papyrus into the incubation room. For Romans, it seems, dreams were had in order that they could be written down. Aristides claims to have written more than 300,000 lines in the dream journal he used as his book's raw material. Scholars later call that journal we will never get to read "the rejected way" of telling the story.[3]

The Tibetan Book of the Dead also provides instruction for interpreting dreams as messages of prognosis. Its authors divine death from dreaming of being surrounded by crows or anguished spirits, or of being dragged along by a crowd of dead people, or of being naked with one's hair cut off. Cancer treatment means I am often half-naked with my hair cut off. I read PubMed instead of my dreams for clues to how long I will live, and the more I read, the more I fear dying somewhere along the path of expensive and diabolical treatments, then for hours these statistics alternate with online shopping, reading wig reviews, dissatisfied. I imagine a thousand fake things on me and a thousand other fake things in me and then a thousand fake things pending and then another thousand fake things forming and another thousand fake things in retreat.

The ancient physician Galen wrote that Aristides was of the rare type whose soul was strong while his body was weak.[4] Aristides continued to write, teach, and speak while "his whole body wasted away." I google my disease and feel alone in the surreality of its quantitative production. Although I have no opinions of the strength of my soul, I am a common type of person, which means I must work for a living, so during my illness I also continue to write, teach, and speak. In the interstices of my to-do list I search for death, desperate for the study that says I will live. I begin to dream of death and know not to obey the night's instructions. I wake up and search for my body's mortal exception. I read the results of a prognosis calculator, LifeMath,[5] then I fall asleep again, dream of death in its curves.

The day I found *it*, I wrote the story I was always writing, the one about how someone and I had been together again, how we shouldn't be, and how I hoped we might finally be able to stop being together soon. We were not happy. We were never able to be together without going to bed. We were never able to go to bed with each other and be happy. We were never able to be happy when not together, and this is why we always found ourselves together, sad, and in bed. We had known each other for years and our knowing each other took the shape of a durable web of *we shouldn't* in which extravagant forms of mutually self-inflicted suffering were caught.

First, there was sex, then the discovery, then there was the escalator ride to the box office for our movie tickets, then I called my doctor for an appointment, then I wrote in my journal how I hoped we might finally be getting closer to not being made miserable by the presence of each other upon the earth. I didn't write down that we had found a thing in my breast or the name of the action movie we went to when we got out of bed.

My fear wasn't of cancer itself, about which I knew almost nothing then. My fear came from a search engine. I was afraid of what Google gave back to me when I entered "breast lump" into it, afraid of the culture of disease as circulated on blogs and on discussion boards, afraid of how people were turned into patients with handles and signatures, agonies, neologisms, and encouragements. Mets. Foobs. NED.[6] I was afraid, on the first day, for my vocabulary.

All that had happened was that I wrote in my journal with precisely avoidant detail, recorded the minor motions of what a person does when she is anxious for a reason she refuses to specify, how I did the laundry, swept the floors, made the beds, swore I'd get over a problematic love, told myself one story so I wouldn't have to tell another.

We are told cancer is an intruder to be fought or an errant aspect of ourselves or an overambitious cell type or an analogy for capitalism or a natural phenomenon with which to live or a certain agent of death. We are told it is in our DNA, or we are told it is in the world, or we are told it is located in the confused admixture of genes and environment that no one can locate or wants to. We are given only the noisy half of probability that its cause is located inside of ourselves and never the quiet part of probability that cancer's source pervades our shared world. Our genes are tested: our drinking water isn't. Our body is scanned, but not our air. We are told it is in the error of our feelings or told it is in the inevitabilities of our flesh. We are told there is a difference between illness and health, between what is acute and what is chronic, between living and dying, too. The news of cancer comes to us on the same sort of screens as the news about elections, in email at the same minute as invitations to LinkedIn. The hash marks of the radiologists are the same as those of the drone pilots. The screen life of cancer is the screen life of all mediated global terror and unreality, too.

Cancer doesn't feel real. Cancer feels like an alien that industrial capitalist modernity has worried into an encounter: mid-astral, semi-sensory, all terrible. Cancer's treatment is like a dream from which we only half-wake to find that half-waking is another chapter in the book of the dream, a dream that is a document and a container for both waking and sleep, any pleasure and all pain, the unbearable nonsense and with it all erupted meaning, every moment of the dream too vast to forget and every recollection of it amnesiac.

The breast surgeon said the greatest risk factor for breast cancer was having breasts. She wouldn't give me the initial results of the biopsy if I was alone. My friend Cara worked for an hourly wage and had no time off without losing out on money she needed to live, so she drove out to the suburban medical office on her lunch break in order that I could get my diagnosis. In the United States, if you aren't someone's child, parent, or spouse, the law allows no one else guaranteed leave from work to take care of you.[7] If you are loved outside the enclosure of family, the law doesn't care how deeply—even with all the unofficialized love in the world enfolding you, if you need to be cared for by others, it must be in stolen slivers of time. As Cara and I sat in the skylit beige of the conference room waiting for the surgeon to arrive, Cara gave me the switchblade she carried in her purse so that I could hold on to it under the table. After all of those theatrical prerequisites, what the surgeon said was what we already knew: I had at least one cancerous tumor, 3.8 centimeters, in my left breast. I handed Cara back her knife damp with sweat. She then went back to work.

The rest of the pathology report came in after I was sent from the surgeon to the oncologist. In Siddhartha Mukherjee's "biography" of cancer, *The Emperor of All Maladies*, it is the Queen of Persia—Atossa—who becomes the iconic breast cancer patient, traveling from 550 B.C. through time in search of treatment. That first time at the oncologist's—also my first time in a waiting room full of chemotherapy patients, none of them royalty—Mukherjee's thought experiment of a fixed aristocratic sufferer, touring fungible medical contexts, became vividly emblematic of cancer culture's myths. Cancer is not a sameness eternalized in an ahistorical body, moving through a trajectory of advancing technological progress.[8] No patient is sovereign, and every sufferer, both those marked by cancer treatment and those marked by the exhausting routine of caring for those with cancer, is also marked by our historical particulars, constellated in a set of social and economic relations.

The history of illness is not the history of medicine—it is the history of the world—and the history of having a body could well be the history of what is done to most of us in the interest of the few.

On a scrap of yellow paper, the oncologist—the one my friends and I later called Dr. Baby because of how much he resembled a cherub—wrote in a childish hand, "hormone receptive positive breast cancer," explaining that there were targeted treatments for it, then crossed it out. Then he wrote, "*Her2* positive breast cancer," explaining that there were targeted treatments for it, then crossed it out. Then he wrote "Triple Negative," and explained that there were no targeted treatments for it. Accounting for between 10 and 20 percent of breast cancers, it has the fewest treatment options and significantly poorer prognoses than others, responsible for a disproportionate number of breast cancer deaths. He said this was the cancer I had. He said the tumor was necrotic, which meant that it was growing so quickly it failed to build infrastructure for itself. He wrote down "85%" for the tumor's growth rate, and I asked him what that meant. He told me that a Ki-67 score of "anything over twenty percent" was highly aggressive.[9] He then said, "Neoadjuvant chemotherapy," which meant "right away."[10] I didn't agree to dissect any nodes or biopsy the other potential areas the doctors feared were tumors: this one certain tumor was bad news enough, and its treatment would be so aggressive I felt like there wasn't any point in a painful intervention to know what else was there.

Something that Mukherjee's book got right was that if the Persian queen Atossa was diagnosed with chemotherapy-resistant triple-negative breast cancer, "her chances of survival will have barely changed."[11] To not submit to chemotherapy was to die, Dr. Baby suggested. To submit to it, I thought, was to feel like dying but possibly to live, or to die from secondary effects rather than primary disease, or to live, finally, almost restored, but not quite. On the way home, the car radio posed a question that I didn't have the power to resolve: *Should I stay or should I go?* But as I moved through the dial, I couldn't find the song with the answer. The staying or going involved the staying or going in this life. Should I live or should I die? But nothing was that frankly posed. As soon as a patient lies down on the exam table, she has laid down her life on a bed of narrowed answers, but the questions are never sufficiently clear.

What will be the outcome of this illness? resembles the questions asked by detectives, art collectors, and graphologists, or anyone who moves some unobvious incidental detail into the heart of a story.[12] Enchantment exists when things are themselves and not their uses. That's why enchantment begins to fade the moment we believe that a collection of cells can predict the agonies of next June. Under the conditions of suspicious interpretation, nothing is ever again as perfect as enchantment was, back when hairs that fell from heads were once records of the beauty of those heads, not soon-to-be-ziplocked evidence of a crime.

After a cancer diagnosis, very little is ever itself again. The nurses give me a glossy binder with a photo of a smiling silver-haired woman on its cover. The title is *Your Oncology Journey*, but I am certain that trip can't be mine. Every step is on the road to Delphi, crowded with divination, every fortune now accompanied by the curse of it-could-be-worse, with the worst being even worse than that. All during, the fortune-tellers never stop offering fortunes and never stop offering along with their fortunes exotic guarantees for or against or faulty reasons why, all of which seem like more lies on lies layered into an increasingly repellent and catastrophic truth of I-can't-know-anything-so-why-try.

Meanwhile, with each step every sensation is as spectacular as a crime scene. No detail is too small to be magnified into the evidence that everything in the world is wrong. And every crime scene of sensation is the future or concurrent scene of uncountable other crimes, some of these crimes in the name of cure and the others in the name of the world as it is, all of them happening all during the investigation, all of them themselves creating more sensation and along with that a spectacle and massacre and interpretive opportunity, layering hurt on hurt, fortune on fortune, lie on lie.

To be diagnosed with cancer right now is not to live in a binder's trajectory: your oncology journey is a lie. "A painting is not," wrote John Cage, "a record of what was said and what the replies were but the thick presence all at once of a naked self-obscuring body of history."[13] To be a cancer patient right now is to exist all at once as the thick presence of the naked self-obscuring history of bodies.

3.

Aelius Aristides called the period of his life in which he lived as an incubant at the temple of Asclepius his *Cathedra*. The visibly dying were never allowed into the temple, nor were the visibly pregnant: birth and death were kept discreetly in structures built in the adjacent territories. The faithful sick passed their time bathing, making burnt offerings, sleeping, waking up, and talking to each other about their dreams. Then they would follow their dreams' prescriptions. The dreams of the incubants were often of two types. The first of these were dreams with instructions that fell inside the boundaries of Roman medical practice—fasting, dietary changes, drugs, phlebotomy, purges—and the other, dreams with prescriptions so wild that the physicians at Pergamum were said to shudder upon hearing them.

Diagnosis has diminished my ability to tell the difference between good advice and empty ideology.[14] Everything I am advised to do in response to the cancer seems, at first, like a symptom of a world that is sick itself. I write in my journal, "the body in the intimacy of the machine," then read on a discussion board that cutting my hair short will make its eventual loss easier to bear. I try to believe this. I usually cut my own, but this time make an appointment at a salon—the Belle Époque—and sit in the elevated chair, saying nothing, while a blond stranger chops my long dark hair above my shoulders. As my hair falls into a pile to be swept up later by a poorly paid assistant with a push broom, I realize then that without ever knowing it I had, at least some years of my life, almost been beautiful and now wouldn't be anymore. I think, too, of how once I always insisted that the best thing about life was that hair grew, which was the simple evidence that nothing stayed the same forever, and therefore proof of the possibilities that the world could change. Now it wasn't just that my hair would fall out, it was that my follicles would die, and painfully, that what once grew would stop growing even as I myself kept living, and everything I once understood about the world as evident would be subject to another proof.

"Variable and therefore miserable condition of man!" wrote the English poet John Donne in his 1624 sickbed masterpiece, *Devotions upon Emergent Occasions*, a prose work written in twenty-three parts over the twenty-three days of what Donne thought was a fatal illness. "This minute I was well, and am ill, this minute."[15]

No one knows you have cancer until you tell them. I take a screen capture of John Donne's first devotion and post it to Facebook: "We study health and we deliberate upon our meats, and drink, and air, and exercises, and we hew, and we polish every stone that goes to that building; and so our health was long and a regular work: but in a minute a cannon batters all."[16]

It gets a lot of likes. Then I follow the other instructions I find on the Internet: tell my mother, tell my daughter, deep clean the kitchen, negotiate with my employer, find someone to watch the cat, go to the thrift store to find clothes that will accommodate my coming chemo port, worry on the phone to my friends that I have no one to take care of me. It is decided without ceremony that the doctors will eventually take my breasts from me and discard them in an incinerator, and because of it, I begin the practice of pretending that my breasts were never there.

A person with aggressive cancer is rarely in a position to reject anyone's prayers, magic, or money. Friends begin an online fund-raiser. Acquaintances give me crystals. On someone's advice, I try past-life regression, where instead of the royalty everyone else seems to be in their earlier incarnations, I am an elderly man with leprosy who is begging, sick and sadder than I ever have been. In another life, I am a child who barely lives and mostly dies. I don't believe in any of this, but it makes sense to me that I've been the greatest possible version of nobody in every possible life.

Ancient temples of healing were built in valleys next to springs and caves. The sick brought the god Asclepius votives of ailing body parts in exchange for healing: sculpted legs, arms, eyeballs. Asclepius's powers were rumored to be so strong he could use the blood of Medusa to raise the dead. Some say that under the grandest of Asclepius's temples was a pit of a thousand snakes. These temple snakes were sometimes let loose among the incubants, who would be pleased by any encounter with them, believing that the slither of a snake over a toe could heal them.

Contemporary oncological images are mostly of faces, and all of them are radiant with multiracial age-spanning happiness. The faces beaming out from cancer's instructional materials bear signs of cancer as social ritual (a bald head, an appropriately colored ribbon) but bear no mark of suffering, not from cancer, but also not from anything else—not work, not racism, not heartbreak, not poverty, not abuse, not disappointment. Our temples collect smiles sanitized from history, every photo of our illnesses a votive of glossy and dubious happiness.

If I were an incubant in the days of Aristides, I'd have to bring a votive of alien math as it caresses deadly inevitability. I didn't feel sick. But this is not quite true. In the weeks between discovering the tumor and the start of chemotherapy, the tumor began to hurt and never stopped, its life making noise against mine. I asked the surgeon if this was because the tumor was growing, and because it was such an aggressive cancer, and she said, *yes, this kind, probably.* I would have known I was sick soon enough. I would have gone to Asclepius bearing a votive of my left breast.

I begin to collect images of Saint Agatha holding her amputated breasts on a platter. Agatha is the patron saint of breast cancer, fires, volcanic eruptions, single women, torture victims, and the raped. She is also the patron saint of earthquakes, because when the torturers amputated her breasts, the ground began to tremble in revenge.

4.

Enchantment is not the same as mystification. One is the ordinary magic of all that exists existing for its own sake, the other an insidious con. Mystification blurs the simple facts of the shared world to prevent us from changing it. Cancer's disenchantments give its mystifications room. I hadn't thought much about breast cancer before I had it, but at first when I did I thought it was simple. I had believed it was no longer very deadly and that its treatment had been made easy, that with breast cancer your life gets a little interrupted but then you get through. Perhaps if I had another cancer this would have been the case, but nothing was easy with my cancer, particularly not finding the truth. All the information seemed designed to make me confused.

There had to be a simple fact, or a set of them, but I could not see the truth with the screen in my face, ardent that somewhere inside my computer, I would find a warrant to live.

My tumor started on a screen, and I returned it there. I entered its precise qualities into the prognostic calculator that promised to display the future in a pictograph. The dead women were represented by forty-eight dark pink frowning faces, the living ones by fifty-two smiling green ones. All of these faces were supposed to, like me, be forty-one years old and with exactly the same version of my disease, but none of these faces, living or dead, said *why* or *when* or *who*.

I didn't know anything about having cancer, but I knew something about how to avoid telling a story. The previous night's dream was another kind of institution—something lit blue, in a glass office building in the sort of city one would find as the backdrop for a television series about lawyers.

Everything about being sick is written in our bodies first and sometimes written in notebooks later. Erotics are rarely allowed in cancer, and this is probably not a novel, but I would rather be Marguerite Duras, to write of love or its disappointments. Once treatment begins, my erotic longing is for assistive devices: a wheelchair and someone to push it, a bedpan and someone to empty it. Then my longing is to spend an hour in consideration of the act of "moving" each time I must move, mentally rehearsing this event of movement, preparing each part of my body that will be required to move and in what relationship with the others, and then to move and to find all the mental preparation had no effect on movement's difficulty. Before I got sick I was strong, but soon to be so weak that to walk short distances, like the six feet from the bed to the bedroom door, left me winded. First a whole life of being appetitive, then to not be able to eat or have sex and to not want to, to not have it matter too much because I also can't without great effort shop for or prepare food or raise my hand to stroke in tenderness the no one that is here; then to not sleep, also, from an exhaustion so fulminating that it is too exhausting for the body to relieve it—and all that time, too, in multifocal pain, which like exhaustion I will write about later, but which will be, to paraphrase Clarice Lispector, like taking a photograph of the scent of a perfume.

Lispector describes her book *Aqua Viva* as "the story of instants that flee like fugitive tracks seen from the window of the train."[17] Aristides begins his *Sacred Tales* with a declaration of the difficulties of writing about the experience of sickness:

> I have never been persuaded by any of my friends, who have asked or encouraged me to speak or write about these things, and so I have avoided the impossible. For it seemed to be the same as if I should swim under water through every sea and next be compelled to render an account of how many waves I encountered, and how I found the sea at each of them, and what it was that saved me.[18]

BIRTH OF THE PAVILION

I am continually beset by the fear that I may
have expressed only a sigh when I thought
I was stating a truth.

—STENDHAL, *On Love*, 1821

communiqué from an exurban satellite clinic of a cancer pavilion named after a financier

Pull your hair out by the handfuls in socially distressing locations: Sephora, family court, Bank of America, in whatever location where you do your paid work, while in conversation with the landlord, at Leavenworth prison, however in the gaze of men. Negotiate for what you need because you will need it now more than ever. If these negotiations fail, yank your hair out of your head in front of who would deny you, leave clumps of your hair in the woods, on the prairies, in QuikTrip parking lots, in front of every bar at which your conventionally feminine appearance earned you and your friends pitchers of domestic beer.

Put your head out the window of the car and let the wind blow the hair off your head. Let your friends harvest locks of your hair to give to other friends to leave in socially distressing locations: to scatter at ports, at national monuments, inside the architecture built to make ordinary people feel small and stupid, to throw against harassers on the streets.

Pull your pubic hair out in clumps from the root and send it in unmarked envelopes to technocrats. Leave your armpit hair at the Superfund site you once lived near, your nose hairs for any human resources officer who denies you leave.

When your eyelashes fall out, send them as a reverse wish to every person who has, at your illness, disappeared. Your hair will fall out onto every surface you come near: it will fall into new alphabets and new words. Read these words to discover the etiology of your illness: If you are lucky you will read another word that means "illness has turned you into an armament." In the bald spots, you will read how to weaponize your dying cells against what you hate and what hates you.

As you see a weapon in your falling hair, also you will see your body as it falls is a weapon, also as it doesn't fall. In this new theory of being a sick person your friend will say that caring for you is now to care for arms. You have turned your room into an armory. Everyone who brings you water or food is also now loading a gun.

1.

The cancer pavilion is a cruel democracy of appearance: the same bald head, the same devastated complexion, the same steroid-swollen face, the same plastic chemotherapy port visible as a lump under the skin. The old seem infantile, the young act senile, the middle-aged find all that is middle-aged about them disappears.

The boundaries of our bodies break. Everything we were supposed to keep inside of us now seems to fall out. Blood from chemotherapy-induced nosebleeds drips on the sheets, the paperwork, the CVS receipts, the library books. We can't stop crying. We emit foul odors. We throw up.

We have poisonous vaginas and poisoned sperm. Our urine is so toxic that the signs in the bathroom instruct patients to flush twice. We do not look like people: we look like people with cancer. We resemble a disease before we resemble ourselves.

Language is no longer compliant to its social function. If we use words it is to approach as a misplaced bomb. Someone mentions something about the weather: in response, an errant phrase from a phantom conversation: "We must learn to accept what we want." Sentences hold out against syntax. Vocabularies re-form into awkward translations of words we once knew or new words we never will. Children who were once taught to speak by their mothers now stare at their sick mothers, who are gesturing like babies learning to talk, unable to recall the word for "television" or the word for "cup."

In the waiting rooms, the labor of care meets the labor of data. Wives fill out their husbands' forms. Mothers fill out their children's. Sick women fill out their own.

I am sick and a woman. I write my own name. I am handed at each appointment a printout from the general database that I am told to amend or approve. The databases would be empty without us.

Receptionists distribute forms, print the bracelets to be read later by scanners held in the hands of other women. The nursing assistants stand in a doorway from which they never quite emerge. They hold these doors open with their bodies and call out patients' names. These women are the paraprofessionals in the thresholds, weighing the bodies of patients on digital scales, taking measurements of vital signs in the staging area of a clinic's open crannies. Then they lead the patient (me) to an examining room and log into the system. They enter the numbers my body generates when offered to machines: how hot or cold I am, the rate at which my heart is beating. Then they ask the question: *Rate your pain on a scale of one to ten?* I try to answer, but the correct answer is always anumerical. Sensation is the enemy of quantification. There is no machine, yet, to which a nervous system can submit sensation to be transformed into a sufficiently descriptive measurement.

Contemporary medicine hyper-responds to the body's unruly event of illness by transmuting it into data. Patients become information not merely via the quantities of whatever emerges from or passes through their discrete bodies, the bodies and sensations of entire populations become the math of likelihood (of falling ill or staying well, of living or dying, of healing or suffering) upon which treatment is based. The bodies of all people are subject to these calculations, but it is women, most often, who do the preliminary work of relocating the nebulousness and uncountablity of illness into medicine's technologized math.

What is your name and birth date? A cancer patient's name, stated by herself, is adjunct to the bar code of her wristband, then the adjunct of whatever substances— vials of drawn blood, the chemotherapy drugs to be infused into her—whose location and identity must be confirmed. Though my bracelet had been scanned for my identity, requiring me to repeat my name is medical information's backup plan: it is the punctum of every transmission of something to or from my body. I might sometimes remember who I am. But repetition is a method of desensitization. To rate your*self* on the scale of 1 to 10? In cancer's medicalized abstraction, I became a *barely*, tertiary to the body's sensations and medicine's informatic systems.

The nurses meet me in the examining room after I have replaced my clothes with a gown. They log into the system. Sometimes my blood has been drawn, and I am allowed to look at a printed page of its ingredients. Each week the blood flows with more or less of one kind of cell or substance than it did the week before. These substances go up or down, determine treatment's future measurement, duration. The nurses ask questions about my experience of my body. They enter the sensations I describe into a computer, clicking on symptoms that have long been given a category and a name and an insurance code.

The word "care" rarely calls to mind a keyboard. The work, often unwaged or poorly paid, of those who perform care (or what is sometimes called "reproductive labor"—reproducing oneself and others as living bodies each day, of feeding, cleaning, tending to, and so on) is what many understand to be that which is the least technological, the most affective and intuitive. "Care" is so often understood as a mode of feeling, neighboring, as it does, love. Care seems as removed from quantification as the cared-for person's sensations of weakness or pain seem removed from statistics class. *I care for you* suggests a different mode of abstraction (that of feeling) than the measurement of the cell division rate of a tumor (that of pathological fact). But strange reversals reveal themselves during serious illness. Or rather, what appears to be reversal becomes clarification. Our once solid, unpredictable, sensing, spectacularly messy and animal bodies submit—imperfectly, but also intensively—to the abstracting conditions of medicine. Likewise, care becomes vivid and material.

The receptionists, nursing assistants, lab technicians, and nurses are not only required to enter the information of my body into the databases, they also have to *care* for me while doing so. In the hospital, my urine is measured and charted by the same person who comforts me with conversation. This is so that painful procedures will become less painful. The workers who check my name twice, scan my medical wristband, and perform a two-person dose-accuracy reinforcement system as they attach chemotherapy drugs to my chest port are the same workers who touch my arm gently when I appear afraid. The worker who draws blood tells a joke. The work of care and the work of data exist in a kind of paradoxical simultaneity: what both hold in common is that they are done so often by women, and like all that has historically been identified as women's work, it is work that can go by unnoticed. It is often noted only when it is absent: a dirty house attracts more attention than a clean one. The background that appears effortless appears only with great effort: the work of care and the work of data are quiet, daily, persistent, and never done. A patient's file is, like a lived-in home, the site of work that lasts the human eternal.

During my treatment for cancer, most of these workers—the receptionists, paraprofessionals, and nurses—have been women. The doctors, who are sometimes women and sometimes men, meet with me at the point of my body's peak quantification. They log into the system, but they type less or sometimes not at all. As their eyes pass over the screen that displays my body's updated categories and quantities, I think of John Donne again: "They have seen me and heard me, arraigned me in these fetters and received the evidence, I have cut up mine own anatomy, dissected myself and they are gone to read upon me."[1]

If it is the women who transmute bodies into data, it is the doctors who interpret the data. The other workers have extracted and labeled me: I have informaticized my own sensation. It is the doctors who read me—or rather, read what my body has become: a patient made of information, produced by the work of women.

In approximately sixty hours, and for the second time, Adriamycin will be infused into my body through a plastic port surgically implanted into my chest and connected to my jugular vein. Adriamycin is named for the Adriatic Sea, near which it was discovered. Its generic name is doxorubicin, a name derived from "ruby" because it is a brilliant and voluptuous red. I like to think of this poison as the ruby of the Adriatic, where I have never been but would like to go, but it is also called "the red devil" and sometimes it is called "the red death," so maybe it should be called *the satanic jewel of mortality on the shores of Venice*, too.

In order to administer the medicine, the oncology nurse, after checking the prescription with a partner, must dress in an elaborate protective costume and slowly, personally, push the Adriamycin through the port in my chest. The medicine destroys tissue if it escapes the veins: it is sometimes considered too dangerous to everyone and everything else to administer by drip. It is rumored, if spilled, to melt the linoleum on a clinic floor. For several days after the drug is administered, my body's fluids will be toxic to other people and corrosive to my body's own tissues. Adriamycin is sometimes fatal to the heart, and has a lifetime limit, of which, by the end of this treatment, I will have reached half.

In the United States, Adriamycin was widely approved for use the year after I was born, 1974, and this means that, including the years spent testing it, its use in cancer patients is older than I am. This is probably the same treatment Susan Sontag was given before she wrote *Illness as Metaphor*, one of the first books someone mails to me when I fall ill. To endure Adriamycin feels like an ancient rite, performed across the decades and on the occasion of many types of cancers as a ritual induction whether a patient needs it or not. Because of how it kills off cells totally in a classic way—turning people bald, making them throw up—its consequences feel like the oncological definitive. Lots of people have cancers that leave few marks on their appearance, but a *cancer victim*—in the cinematic sense—is a person who has had this kind of chemotherapy. That my treatment begins with it is a clear sign of how little progress has been made.

Treatment with Adriamycin can cause leukemia, heart failure, organ failure, and will almost certainly cause me infertility and infection. Because, like many chemotherapy drugs, Adriamycin is a generalist in its destructions, it is also toxic to the central nervous system, and my mitochondria will begin to react to it three hours after its administration. This will continue for up to twenty-seven hours, but the damage cascades beyond treatment, is often sustained for years. As I sit in the infusion chair, the white and gray matter of my brain will begin to diminish. There is no particular way to know how this will change me: the brain damage from chemotherapy is cumulative and unpredictable. Although the drug has been in use for half a century, because it does not cross the blood-brain barrier, doctors sometimes did not believe patients about its cognitive effects, or when they heard these, they sometimes minimized the patients' complaints as other kinds of cancer-related unhappiness.

MRIs of others who have had this chemotherapy for breast cancer suggest damage to the visual cortex, "significantly reduced activation of the left middle dorsolateral prefrontal cortex and premotor cortex," and "significantly reduced left caudal lateral prefrontal cortex activation, increased perseverative errors, and reduced processing speed."[2] Patients report that they lose the ability to read, to recall words, to speak fluently, to make decisions, and to remember. Some lose not just their short-term memories, but their episodic ones: that is, they lose memory of their lives.

These effects, of which Dr. Baby informed me casually only as he was escorting me to my first infusion of chemotherapy, are said to be inevitable. Nothing can be done, *Your Oncology Journey* tells me, except to endure one's brain-damaged life with "good humor." The effects can last throughout treatment, or for one year, or grow worse in the years after treatment, last for ten years or more.[3]

Sick people sit in waiting rooms, and if they recline, it is temporarily, and if they are too weak to sit, they sit despite this, their heads slumped against their necks. No matter how sick they are, the sick who are treated at the cancer pavilion do not spend most of their time there: they are sick at work and sick at home or sick at school or sick in the grocery store or sick in the DMV or sick in their automobiles or on buses. Some are wheeled in by their children or partners or volunteers or friends, then wheeled out again into cars taking them to apartments or houses, all of which, like cancer treatment, must be paid for.

The word "clinic" is derived from the Greek *clīnicus*, meaning "of or pertaining to a bed." The word "pavilion," on the other hand, is intended for an entirely different structure, suggestive of jousts and battlefields. A pavilion is a place for generals and kings, almost always temporary and luxurious architecture erected for the purposes of the powerful, adjacent to something else—in cancer's case, adjacent to all the rest of what we call *life*.

The philosopher Michel Foucault wrote a famous book about the spatial arrangement of illness called *The Birth of the Clinic*, but I can't find a book called *The Birth of the Pavilion*. It seems impossible that a cancer pavilion could have a mother. In the large and bustling space in which my cancer treatment is administered I have never seen a bed.

Activity inside the pavilion is transient, abstracted, impermanent, dislocated. The sick and the partners, children, parents, friends, and volunteers who care for them are kept in circulation from floor to floor, chair to chair. The doctors are assigned a rotation of offices and outposts, and in order to find out where yours is each day, you have to call ahead.

Cancer treatment appears organized for the maximum profit of someone—not the patients—which means cancer patients are kept in maximum circulation at a maximum rate. Foucault wrote, "The clinic should have had only one direction—from top to bottom, from constituted knowledge to ignorance."[4] The pavilion, on the other hand, is a tangle of directions. Money and mystification, not knowledge or ignorance, are its cardinal points.

Scientists discovered the drug known as *the red devil* near Castel del Monte, built by the Holy Roman Emperor Frederick II in Italy in the 1240s. The castle had neither a moat nor a drawbridge, so few believe it was ever used as a fortress. It never was completely finished, so some people think it was only used as a temporary lodge. The castle was built in a rare octagonal shape, and later it became a prison, then a refuge during the plague. Then the Bourbons stripped out its marble. Then the scientists harvested its dirt. Taking the castle soil back to Milan, they found *Streptomyces peucetius*, the bright red bacteria from which my treatment came. Adriamycin is an anthracycline, which means it blocks an enzyme called topoisomerase II. By blocking this enzyme, the drugs inhibit the rapid proliferation of cells—many of the cells we need, but ideally also the cells we don't.[5]

I was given the Adriamycin with cyclophosphamide, a drug approved for use in 1959, in a common treatment combination called dense-dose AC chemo. Cyclophosphamide is a medicalized form of a chemical weapon already developed by Bayer under the name LOST.

Mustard gas, as it is also known, has always done its worst as an incapacitant rather than a killer, but it can kill a person, too. During World War I, LOST filled the trenches with brilliant yellow plumes.[6] During cancer, it comes in plastic pouches, and no one in the pavilion speaks frankly about what it is. Outlawed as a weapon in 1925, it is a form of slow obliteration that lives on only in chemotherapy and, after that, as its own consequences: infection, infertility, cancer, cognitive loss. In chemotherapy, as in war, when you are being exposed to cyclophosphamide, it is advisable that you have someone to hold your hand.

Although four dense-dose rounds of old-fashioned drugs effectively eliminated many parts of me, some of them still half-dead, neither of these drugs appeared to significantly reduce my tumor. After we were done with all that cellular annihilation, my own semi-annihilation was obvious but my tumor remained intact. It remained as the full measure of shadow inside the radiance of the screen.

A patient is a system-containing object within a series of interlocking systems full of other system-containing objects. As an object, a patient can function (comply) or break (cease compliance). "To cease compliance" can mean "to display any potential for agency"—to ask, perhaps, too many questions, to bring in conflicting research, to refuse a procedure, to consistently show up to the waiting room at least fifteen minutes late.

If I die from this cancer, I tell my friends, cut my corpse into pieces and send my right thigh to Cargill, my left hand to Apple, my ankles to Procter and Gamble, my forearm to Google.[7]

A cancer patient might believe that to cease compliance with treatment is a revolt against how the system of medicine has objectified them, but they are probably wrong. A patient's noncompliance is, for that system, not evidence that a person exists as autonomous and thoughtful and capable of intelligent nonconsent, but it is viewed as interference of other systems—contaminating ones such as "misinformation" or "superstition."

The system of medicine is, for the sick, a visible scene of action, but beyond it and behind it and beneath it are all the other systems, *family race work culture gender money education*, and beyond those is a system that appears to include all the other systems, the system so total and over-whelming that we often mistake it for the world.

To become a cancer patient is to become a system-containing object inside another system that only partially allows the recognition of the rest of the systems in which one is a node and also almost wholly obscures the heaviest system of the arrangement of the world as it is, which hangs around, too, in the object that contains a system (by which I mean "me") as part of the problem in the first place, requiring our latent unhealth just as it profits from our active one.

This system we mistake for everything resides in a system-containing object like a tumor inside a system-containing object like a cancer patient who is a system-containing object inside a clinic, all of it also containing these systems of history.

Then there are the traces of that grand and easy-to-mistake-for-everything system, a system we mistake as forever and unchangeable and without remedy and unfair, too, how it resides outside of that patient, both in a close way that she can see how it hurts her and in a faraway she must squint at, barely able to make out its recognizable shapes.

Then people leave, friends drop off, lovers abscond with all possibility of you ever again being fond of them, colleagues avoid you, your rivals are now unimpressed, your Twitter followers unfollow. To the people who have left you, it is possible you are either the most object-like of all possible objects (that you are to someone a thing to be discarded like trash) or the most human that you can be in the situation of this illness (for how strongly, on being discarded, you feel forlorn). Or, as you have learned that anything is possible during catastrophic illness, you could be the most human and the most object all at once.

The ones who have abandoned you, who—now that you are sick—have ceased to speak to you or come around or just say outright that they can't handle it, say that your illness is, as they say, "too difficult" for them, have a hand at creating your existence, at least partially, as someone who will always, at least in part, stay well. To them you are static and permanent. The people who left won't watch you suffer or diminish, so you are, by their actions, kept forever as you were at the moment of diagnosis. You remain vibrant and unaltered in their memories: your hair is thick, your mind is lively, and your eyelashes are long and falling against your flushed cheeks. The abandoners are the people who never have to see you as anything but you.

To yourself, who has not yet developed the consciousness required of your way of life as an object, the abandonment causes you to feel less human mostly in the manner of feeling entirely like an animal. You feel like the kind of animal who is melancholy and looks at any object and wishes to be it instead of yourself, wishes to be a chandelier, maybe, or a silver-plated fork or a wall-mounted machete, wishes to be anything (a bench, the broken heel of a shoe, a locust shell, a flashlight without batteries, a book about ships, a crack in the floorboard, an oak leaf in the gutter, a scalpel, a particle, an attic, a big-box store) but a sick and abandoned animal, wishes to be anything in the world but that which was once loved and now is left alone.

In the week before chemotherapy, it is like preparing for a winter storm, or a winter storm and a houseguest, or a winter storm, a houseguest, and the birth of a child; also, maybe it is as if preparing for all of these and a holiday, a virus, and a brief but intense episode of depression, all while also suffering the effects of the previous storm, houseguest, birth, holiday, virus, and depression.

The day before chemotherapy, a friend arrives from someplace I would rather be—California or Vermont or two different towns named Athens or New York or Chicago. Then it is exactly as it is: as if a friend has arrived from far away. On that day, I do everything to look healthy so that my friend will praise the skillfulness of my camouflage, its materials purchased at Wigs.com, CVS, and Sephora. On the day before chemotherapy, we don't speak of chemotherapy any more than is necessary for the practical exchange of information, like what time to set the alarm and the best route to the pavilion. We pass our time as friends would, roasting vegetables and listening to music and speaking excitedly of other friends or ideas or political events.

The day of chemotherapy we wake up early and arrive at least fifteen minutes late. We predict how well the treatment will go by what song is on the car radio: "Bohemian Rhapsody" (not so good), TLC's "Waterfalls" (better). Chemotherapy, like most medical treatments, is boring. Like death, it is a lot of waiting for your name to be called. It is also waiting while the potential for panic and pain hangs around, too, waiting for its name to be called. In this it is like war. The aesthetics of chemotherapy appear to have been decided by no one. That makes them like everything ideological. Later we begin to understand the costumes, machines, sounds, rituals, and architectures.

A nurse in a hazmat suit inserts a large needle into my plastic subdermal port. First things are drawn from me, then things are flushed in and out of me, then things drip into me. For each of these things that drip into me, I must say my own name and when I was born.

Of the many drugs that I am infused with, some of them are drugs with familiar, clear-cut effects: Benadryl, steroids, Ativan. I should know how these feel, but in this context, they never feel like themselves. Instead, they combine with the chemotherapy drugs into a new feeling, each type of chemotherapy mixing with its additives into a unique mush of hybrid lack of clarity.

I was once a prompt person, now I am always late. I was once a person who reacted strongly to a cup of coffee, now I am a person who behaves demi-unreactively to the sludge of substances inside me. I explain to my friend as I am being infused, "They are giving me all the drugs, every last one of them." The oncology nurse agrees, "Yes, we are. We are giving her all the drugs."

I try to be the best-dressed person in the infusion room, wrap myself up in thrift-store luxury and pin it together with a large gold brooch in the shape of a horseshoe. The nurses always praise the way I dress. I need that. Then they infuse me with a platinum agent, among other things, and I am a person in thrift-store luxury with platinum running through her veins.

After the infusion is over, I sit up until I fall over. I don't give up until I give up, try to win all the board games, remember all the books any of us have read, go out if I can, try to flirt and gossip and analyze into the night. Terrible things are happening in my body. Sometimes I will say it to my companions: "Terrible things are happening inside of me." Finally, forty or forty-eight or sixty hours later, I can't move and there is nothing to take for the pain, but trying to be obedient to medicine and polite to my friends, I take something for the pain.

Then there is the slow drip of circumstance and effect—a new problem or several each day for seven days or fourteen of them. I begin to feel a flicker of ambition again: first alien, then increasingly like myself—or myself, but disabled, but never predictably disabled, only as if a cloud of disability floats around my body, landing in one system or location or the next and then finding another, quickly, as soon as I have compensated for it.

I have always wanted to do everything and know everything and be everywhere, and because of this, I feel left out, captive, bored. But mostly I feel asynchronous—both hurried and left behind. Time, apart from pain, work, family, mortality, medicine, information, aesthetics, history, truth, love, literature, and money, is cancer's other big problem.

2.

At the fullest expression of its treatment, breast cancer is near total strike: striking hair, striking eyelashes, striking eyebrows, striking skin, striking thought, striking language, striking feeling, striking vigor, striking appetite, striking eros, striking maternity, striking productivity, striking immune system, negated fertility, negated breasts.

Self-manage, the boss that is everyone says: *work harder, stay positive, draw on eyebrows, cover your head with a wig or colorful scarf, insert teardrop- or half-a-globe-shaped silicone under your scarred skin and graft on prosthetic nipples or tattoo trompe-l'oeil ones in pubescent pink or have flaps of fat removed from your back or belly and joined to your chest, exercise when tired, eat when repulsed by food, go to yoga, do not mention death, take an Ativan, behave normally, think of the future, cooperate with the doctors, attend "look good feel better" for your free high-quality makeup kit,*[8] *run a 5K, whether-or-not-to-wear-a-wig-during-sex is a question the book says to ask your husband, "one family member at a time" says the sign on the way to the infusion room, the pink ribbon on the for-sale sign of the mansion.*

The broad hand of cliché helps out with painful humiliations. Also useful are contradictory unspecifics, as if what actually happens can be unfelt by remaining wrapped up in the padding of being confused.

People with breast cancer are supposed to be ourselves as we were before, but also better and stronger and at the same time heart-wrenchingly worse. We are supposed to keep our unhappiness to ourselves but donate our courage to everyone. We are supposed to, as anyone can see in the YouTube videos, dance toward our mastectomies, or, as in *Sex and the City*, stand up with Samantha in the ballroom and throw off our wigs while a banqueting crowd roars with approval. We are supposed to, as Dana does in *The L Word*, pick ourselves up out of dreary self-pity and look stylish on the streets in our headscarves. If we die later, as Dana does, we are supposed to know our friends will participate in a fundraising athletic event and take a minute, before moving on to other episodes, to remember that we once lived.

We are supposed to be legible as patients and illegible as our actual selves while going to work and taking care of others as our actual selves now with the extra work of the false heroics of legibility as a disease: every patient a celebrity survivor, smiling before the surgery and smiling after, too, bald and radiant and funny and productively exposed. We are supposed to, as the titles of the guide-books instruct, be *feisty, sexy, thinking, snarky* women, or girls, or ladies, or whatever. Also, as the T-shirts for sale on Amazon suggest, we are always supposed to be able to tell cancer "you messed with the wrong bitch."

In my case, however, cancer messed with the right bitch.

I know the point of a test designed so everyone will fail is that no one will pass that test. Then we all feel like fail-ures, but each of us thinks we have failed alone.

Some of us prefer to take the form of background noise, wearing a wig and refusing legibility's grosser narrative.

I like wigs. I wear wigs. People I like wear wigs. Dolly Parton wears wigs. Beyoncé wears wigs. Enlightenment philosophers wore wigs. Drag queens, Egyptian prin-cesses, and grandmothers wear wigs. Medusa wore a wig made of snakes.

If you hadn't consented to treatment, the bad feelings would probably have come later. But you did, so the bad feelings are happening now. The only certain universe of a Thursday morning is sterile, hypothetical, and smelling of Purell. A sparrow flies head-on into the window of the pavilion, recovers, then does it again. Everything seems decorated as a protest against interesting. The poet Juliana Spahr has come to visit from California, and she and I fill out prayer cards in the lobby and slide them through the slit cut in the gift-wrapped shoe box: *Please pray*, we write, *for American poetry*.

After chemotherapy on Thursday, I come back to the clinic on Friday for a blood panel and Neulasta—a synthetic protein designed to stimulate the production of white blood cells and ward off infection. At the time of my treatment, each Neulasta shot costs seven thousand dollars, and I get the shot while dressed in my regular aesthetic resistance: Chagall-blue tights, blond wig, a persimmon-colored vintage coat, and—because of my failing immune system—a thin paper mask.

How to stay safe in cancer's pastel-colored danger? You can't retreat into yourself for safety from what is inside yourself or run from yourself for safety from yourself. You can't fight what is in you outright, as one might against an attacker or a wild beast. If you do, *joke's on you*, you are fighting yourself, like when the older kids took hold of your arm and punched your own face with it, forcing you to hit yourself while they repeated "quit hitting yourself" until you cried. When you have cancer, you have to learn to understand what is growing inside you as that which is both yourself and not yourself, as yourself and a thing that, if all goes well, will be taken out of you, too. Self-love under these conditions appears to require you to love the cancer in yourself and to hate it as a threat to yourself, too.

"Fuck cancer"[9] is always the wrong slogan if for no other reason than that the cancer is your own body growing inside you, but also because "cancer" is a historically specific, socially constructed imprecision and not an empirically established monolith. This whole time I've been writing about cancer, I've been writing about something that scientists agree doesn't quite exist, at least not as one unified thing. *Fuck white supremacist capitalist patriarchy's ruinous carcinogenosphere* would be a lot better, but it is a difficult slogan to fit on a hat. The world is guaranteed to change, as everything does, but the sickness inside you could last forever, becoming more of itself while you become less. But if you begin to accept your illness, or even to love it, you worry that you might want to keep it around. You think, when you feel bad, that you will never long for it, but in truth you do, since it provides such clear instruction for existing, brings with it the sharpened optics of life without futurity, the purity of the double vision of any life lived on the line.

3.

In the cancer pavilion, disobedience is dangerous, but so is going along. A patient must adopt a discipline of following instruction in order not to mess up the whole careful process, but doctors can be tired, imprecise, or even prejudiced and incorrigible. Nurses are mostly geniuses, but it feels dangerous to be obedient to doctors, some of whom don't seem to know what they are doing. They grow attached to you and think they know best, or sometimes act petty and vengeful when you ask them a challenging question. If you were ever a rebellious teenager, it becomes too easy to mistake one for a dad.

I begin to think that I have to leave my first oncologist—the one we call Dr. Baby—because, despite its being the standard of care, the treatment he is giving me doesn't seem to work. I bring in studies, I bring in friends, I bring in arguments, I lose sleep. He is good at his job. He makes phone calls, he casts doubt on studies, he brings his best arguments, he tries to persuade my friends. I feel like I am fighting for my life against a putto—a decorative Renaissance cherub. My friends don't know who to believe about this question of my treatment: me, the chemo-damaged *dérangée* spending drug-hazed nights on PubMed, or Dr. Baby, a bald, middle-aged man who wears slip-on clogs because, as he tells us, it takes too much energy to tie shoelaces. Dr. Baby and I quarrel about treatment, but he also explains that he owns a pair of loafers he could wear but that it is too much effort to reach to the top of his closet to get them. The friend who accompanied me to that particular exam said that Dr. Baby on shoes is irrefutable evidence that life is governed by a chance machine.

I like Dr. Baby, of course, and am certain that Dr. Baby cares about me, but not enough to be brave in the way I need him to be. Dr. Baby is making the decisions he believes are best for me, saying that a more aggressive treatment holds too great a risk for a younger patient because of its debilitating future effects. I tell him that to not offer the most aggressive treatment is too great a risk for a young patient because the survival numbers for the standard-of-care treatment are not acceptable. I do not want to die, I tell him. I still have a lot left to do. It is precisely because I still need time, I plead, that I will do anything to live.

My friend Cara has my back. She narrows her eyes and asks him: "What's the worst that can happen?"

Dr. Baby, after listing the disabling long-term side effects, says to Cara, "She could die." Then he says, distraught enough that we believe him, "I've seen people die of chemotherapy." Oncologists, too, fear oncology.

I go to another oncologist for a second opinion. She is a specialist in my cancer. It has been suggested to me that the regimen she prescribes for her patients, in furtherance of her research, is unusually aggressive and controversial. I don't care because I want to live. Dr. Baby appears upset after I make an appointment with her, and after that, he goes from someone who used to call me just to see how I was feeling to someone who won't talk to me even as we sit in the same room. The new oncologist says, upon hearing the facts of my triple negative's specific subtype, that I am correct, that I have read the studies correctly, that the treatment I am asking for is indeed the one she believes will work. I become her patient.

She is correct and I am correct, but Dr. Baby is also correct. The new treatment is disabling, not just during, but for years after. Even by the extreme standards of chemotherapy, it feels like too much. This new oncologist can barely remember my name, has none of Dr. Baby's befuddled charm or intensity of feeling. But within days of the first infusion of the drug combination I was sure I needed, the tumor, which had been a nagging, terrifying, unshrinking pain in my breast for the duration of chemotherapy, finally ceases to hurt.

Someone once said that choosing chemotherapy is like choosing to jump off a building when someone is holding a gun to your head. You jump out of fear of death, or at least a fear of the painful and ugly version of death that is cancer, or you jump from a desire to live, even if that life will be for the rest of its duration a painful one.

There is a choice, of course, and you make it, but the choice never really feels like yours. You comply out of a fear of disappointing others, a fear of being seen as deserving of your suffering, a hope that you could again feel healthy, a fear that you will be blamed for your own dying, a hope that you can put it all behind you, a fear of being named as the person who cannot cheerfully submit to every form of self-preservative self-destruction written in the popular instructions. You comply from ritual obedience, as when the teacher hands out exams, or the bailiff says "All rise," or the minister entreats a prayer, or the cops shout "Move along." You comply from hope that obedience now will result in years in which you can disobey later. You comply because the only other option might be to drink carrot juice and die of your own cellular proliferation, refusing to admit your own mortal vulnerabilities, pinning heartbreaking notes about spontaneous remission around your room.

You must have a desire to live, but it is also necessary to believe that you are a person worth keeping alive. Cancer requires painful, expensive, environmentally harmful, extractive medicine. My desire to survive means I still can't bring myself to unravel survival's ethics. One of the chemotherapy drugs with which I was treated, cyclophosphamide, passes into the urine only partially diluted, is only partially removed by water treatment methods, and lasts in the common water supply for four hundred to eight hundred days.[10] Another, carboplatin, is described in its manufacturer's information sheet as having the "environmental fate" of accumulating in aquatic environments, where it lingers but no one yet knows what damage it does. The Himalayan yew tree, from which one of my chemotherapy drugs is harvested, has been endangered since 2011.[11] Cancer spending was $130 billion in 2017, greater than the GDP of more than a hundred countries.[12] The cost of one chemotherapy infusion was more money than I had then earned in any year of my life.

My problem is that I wanted to live millions of dollars' worth but could never then or now answer why I deserved the extravagance of this existence, why I consented to allow the marketplace to use as its bounty all of my profitable troubles. How many books, to pay back the world for my still existing, would I have to write?

And after treatment, when my body was wrecked, when my body was like a car with parts that kept falling off, when I failed at, as U.S. disability law calls it, "basic activities of daily living," I wondered how all those dollars had passed through my body and I was still left in such bad shape. If I calculated the cost of each breath I took after this cancer, I should breathe out stock options. My life was a luxury good, but I was corroded, I was mutilated, I was uncertain. I was not okay.

__ THE SICKBED

Miserable and (though common to all) inhuman
posture where I must practice my lying in
the grave by lying still and not practice my
resurrection by rising any more!
—JOHN DONNE, *Devotions upon Emergent*
   Occasions, 1623

1.

Sometimes the thought of dying young is more than the punk romance of a person who can't handle an imagined getting old. Once we were teenagers, expecting to die by twenty-eight, and if that didn't work, by forty. Then forty came, its most discernible loss that of any desire for dying early, *live-fast-die-young* the refrain of those who didn't understand a person could mess around with living fast and also slow down as necessary later, could die old and interesting and with each other.

Before you have a chance to cancel the invitation, though, what you only kind of desired in the first place shows up, offers you the preservative honor of dying fuckable in that famous way that people think they love. You could, as a guy in a band once advised you, *always leave them wanting*. You could die before almost anyone you loved did, could be spared grief, global warming, and the collapse of Social Security.

Biography in that case becomes a logic a person can no longer recognize of a form of being that can't exist. It's iconography, not biography, that would offer the Hail

Mary radiance of what it meant to have lived, the newly arrived guest of maybe-dying-early leaning over to whisper in your ear a flattery about hagiography, too, something about how to check out now would make you static, enduring, and inculpable. You could die, if not saintly, at least without the burden of further moral error.

But dead women can't write. And as John Donne wrote in his poem "The Blossom," meaning something else, "A naked thinking heart, that makes no show, / Is to a woman"—by which I mean me—"but a kind of ghost."[1]

Once my hair is gone, once I can no longer taste my food, once I have passed out while shopping for a bread knife in IKEA, once the ex-lovers have all visited to make one last attempt to get me in bed, once the generous humiliations of crowd-sourced charity have assured me months of organic produce, I have become a patient. The old ways are through. Any horizon is made of medicine. Any markers of specific identity beyond "the sick" and "the healthy" become from another era. Cancer mediates all.

Every movie I watch now is a movie about an entire cast of people who seem to not have cancer, or at least this is, to me, its plot. Any crowd not in the clinic is a crowd that feels curated by alienation, all the people everywhere looking robust and eyelashed and as if they have appetites for dinner and solid plans for retirement. I am marked by cancer, and I can't quite remember what the markers are that mark us as who we are when we are not being marked by something else.

Yet I know I existed before I was ill. I kept journals, so have proof. On the first day of 2014, the year in which I will fall ill, I am forty years old, work for a living teaching art students, and have a daughter in eighth grade. We live in a two-bedroom apartment in suburban Kansas City for which I pay around $850 a month. According to my journals, where I dutifully record each day's mundane details, I am wearing an oversized moth-eaten red cashmere sweater that I bought from the Salvation Army, and I seem to have a slight cold. I write that I am optimistic about starting out the new year with a virus. It is as if the old year is being burned out of me through fever and the new one will come in renewed because any illness that doesn't kill you sets you on fire and then you start over, just like that. I am awaiting the next day's delivery of a vintage Queen Anne–style four-poster bed I bought for $280 at a consignment shop. Twenty-six weeks into owning it, the week after my forty-first birthday, it becomes my sickbed—the most tragic piece of furniture I will ever own.

There is no more tragic piece of furniture than a bed, how it falls so quickly from the place we make love to the place we might die in. It is tragic, too, for how it falls so quickly from the place where we sleep to the place where we think ourselves mad. The bed where anyone makes love is also—and too clearly for anyone stuck there because of illness—the grave, as John Donne described it, from which they might never rise.

In vertical life, when you are well or mostly and walking around, pretending to be, the top of your head is the space that the heavens touch. The total area of the top of you is pretty small. You are only moderately airy, then, and your eyes, rather than gazing up, gaze outward at the active world, and it is to this you are mostly reacting. And it is mostly during the night, during dreams, that imagining becomes temporarily expansive and the ceiling air spreads over you, or at least this was, in those days, one magic theory I conjured in bed to explain the relationship of posture to thought.

When you are sick and horizontal, the sky or skyish air of what is above you spreads all over your body, the increased area of airy intersection leads to a crisis of excessive imagining. All that horizontality invites a massive projecting of cognitive forms. When you are so often lying down, you are also so often looking up.

A sick person in bed is the ward of love, if she is lucky, and the orphan of action, even if she is not. All the accumulated gorgeousness of life in bed can be eclipsed by gravity there, and dreams, too, become occluded by pain. Every pleasure of a bed can, during illness, disappear behind fresh architectures of worry.

Harriet Martineau wrote in her 1844 book *Life in the Sick-Room*, "Nothing is more impossible to represent in words . . . than what it is to lie on the verge of life and watch, with nothing to do but to think, and learn from what we behold."[2]

Virginia Woolf's mother, Julia Stephen, also wrote a treatise on sickrooms. In this 1883 work, she instructed caregivers that while the patient in a sickbed may appear to have "absurd" fancies, these are heightened perceptions of the real, a result of the "delicately organized" minds of the very ill, "whose senses have become so acute through suffering."[3]

In John Donne's *Devotions upon Emergent Occasions*, there is a virtuosic enactment of this kind of heightening, an instruction manual from the platform of feeling like hell. Illness can bring thought to that newly exposed mega-cosmos of our senses. Donne wrote:

"Man consists of more pieces, more parts, than the world; than the world doth, nay than the world is. And if those pieces were extended, and stretched out in man as they are in the world, man would be the giant, and the world the dwarf; the world but the map, and the man the world. If all the veins in our bodies were extended to rivers, and all the sinews to veins of mines, and all the muscles that lie upon one another, to hills, and all the bones to quarries of stones, and all the other pieces to the proportion of those which correspond to them in the world, the air would be too little for this orb of man to move in, the firmament would be but enough for this star; for, as the whole world hath nothing, to which something in man doth not answer, so hath man many pieces of which the whole world hath no representation."[4]

A well person's astral projection remains mostly atmospheric, but the deeply ill person in pain, in order to escape it, can sprint away from the pain-husk of the failing body and think themselves into a range beyond range. When pain is so vast, it makes it hard to remember history or miles per hour, which should make the sickbed the incubator for almost all genius and nearly most revolution.

Illness vivifies the magnitude of the body's parts and systems. In the sickbed, the sick disassemble and this disassembly crowds a cosmos, organs and nerves and parts and aspects announcing themselves as unfurling particulars: a malfunctioning left tear duct—a new universe; a dying hair follicle—a solar system; that nerve ending in the fourth toe of the right foot—now eviscerating under chemotherapy drugs—a star about to collapse.

All that time lying down can also bring about the microscopic practice of worry. In the sickbed, illness also illuminates smallness, shabbiness, self-absorption, inconsequence, personal finance, home economics, the social order. Virginia Woolf's mother understood how the small was the great agonist to the ill: "Among the number of small evils which haunt illness, the greatest, in the misery which it can cause, though the smallest in size, is crumbs. The origin of most things has been decided on, but the origin of crumbs in bed has never excited sufficient attention among the scientific world."[5]

Being sick makes excessive space for thinking, and excessive thinking makes room for thoughts of death. But I was always starving for experience, not its cessation, and if the experience of thought was the only experience my body could give me beyond the one of pain, opening myself to wild, deathly thinking had to be allowed. *Don't try to make me*, I warned my friends in a set of emailed instructions, *stop thinking about death.*

In 1621, two years before the December that John Donne fell ill and wrote his sickbed masterpiece, an anonymous Flemish painter painted his or her own. *Young Woman on Her Death Bed* is rare in the tradition of European sickbed paintings in that it is, like actually dying young, actually terrifying. The young woman's skin is waxen, her eyes unfocused, her posture cramped and scared, her hands inert and curled like claws. Her surroundings are fine—smooth linens and velvets, coordinated wallpaper, too—but all the comfort in the world cannot be a comfort in the face of that.

The death of Cleopatra is a better look. She died, according to Wikipedia, on "August 12, aged thirty-nine years, wearing her most beautiful garments, her body arrayed on a golden couch and the emblems of royalty in her hands." In the paintings, Cleopatra is almost always draped over a bed or chaise as if waiting for a lover. Her breast—usually the left one—is exposed, troubled by a slender asp her own hand has guided voluptuously toward her nipple. In Greek tragedy, too, women died only where they slept, made love, and gave birth. As the classicist

Nicole Loraux writes about women's tragic deaths, "Even when a woman kills herself like a man, she nevertheless dies in her bed, like a woman."[6]

No one really knows how Cleopatra killed herself. Her contemporaries' guesses were a snake or two snuck into a basket of figs or flowers, a poisoned hairpin, or a deadly salve. According to Plutarch, Octavian preferred the asp theory, which has had an enduring sex appeal, and depicted this in his triumphal procession: "an effigy of the dead Cleopatra upon a couch was carried by, so that in a way she, too . . . was a part of the spectacle and a trophy."[7]

The anonymous young woman in the anonymously painted Flemish painting is, in her unsexy suffering, no trophy, and in every way an antidote to an early death's seductions. As the painter Marlene Dumas wrote of first seeing Goya's *Fates*, "I covered my mouth as if to prevent the devil from entering."[8]

I was alone in the hospital, and the call button had fallen onto the floor where I couldn't reach it. I wasn't able to climb out of bed, but I could see that someone had put a sticker of a Disney prince on the call button I needed, a joke that went: "someday my prince will come."

"Promise when I am ill, you will take me out back and shoot me," a person at work said. Sometimes people told me, "I would rather die than . . ."—the ellipsis to be filled in with how they would rather be dead than do what I must to live.

The administrator of the breast cancer fetish page—one that gathers photo galleries of fair-skinned young starlets and invents fictional erotic accounts of their breast cancer diagnosis, treatment, and outcomes—has written this: "Thinking about a gorgeous, perfect woman developing a cancerous lump, and it destroying her body and her life, elicits such sorrow and emotion from me that the reaction actually causes sexual stimulation." It goes on: "Now picture them, alone or with a lover, undressing and displaying their beautiful perfect bodies. Now imagine a hand, hers or a lover's, moving over one of her perfect breasts—and discovering a lump. Picture the fear, the shock, and the despair the girls would feel, so young, so perfect, and so filled with cancer in their breasts."

"To look these things squarely in the face would need the courage of a lion tamer; a robust philosophy; a reason rooted in the bowels of the earth," wrote Virginia Woolf in "On Being Ill," an essay in which she claims there is no great literature about being ill.[9] The claim that there is no great literature about being ill is a claim made in almost all great literature about being ill.

On good days, I visit the art museum to look at an 1859 painting by Thomas Couture called *The Illness of Pierrot*. In it, the sick young clown is dressed in white and sinking into his bed. One of Pierrot's fellow clowns, Harlequin, has turned his own face to the wall in a posture of grief. An elderly woman leans expectantly toward the clown in the sickbed. A physician in Enlightenment clothes looks away from the patient, crosses his own stocking-covered legs, reaches his hand toward the clown to feel the pulse. The sick clown was once the life of the party, at least that's what the empty wine bottles near him suggest, but now he is half lost in his linens and not to be helped by the physician who won't look directly at him or the friend who won't stop grieving or the elderly woman who looks but won't touch. Some days I think Pierrot the clown will die, and some days I am certain he will get better, but every time I visit, he seems never to have left his bed. It's a problem with art that sick Pierrot always stays sick.

Only certain kinds of sick people make it into art. There are almost never any sick in humble beds, unless these are the gorgeously humble beds of artists, and no bed on earth is as humble as the other places people are left to be ill and die. I've never seen a painting of an incarcerated woman sick from breast cancer hanging on the wall of the Louvre. I've never seen one of a sick person in a car in a rural emergency room parking lot on the walls of the Met, or a sculpture of a homeless encampment tent at the Vatican, or an installation of a suicide-inducing Foxconn factory in the Uffizi.

I've also never seen a sickbed scene from the point of view of the person in it. A problem with a sickbed scene as painted by the sick person herself is that it would have to be painted on a canvas with no edges, to be too small to measure, to be too large to contain. It would happen outside of time, happen inside of history, exempt the present from the linear, rearrange substance so that blankness is an element, rearrange aesthetics so that the negative is almost all. That kind of painting would be hard to make.

2.

Doing the dishes is not like freedom. Freedom is whatever we notice because it isn't like doing the dishes. The ordinary is ordinary because it ordinarily repeats: *taking care* lacks freedom's entertainments and its exceptions.

For any author of doing the dishes, the best part of the story would be the story of missing out on everything else while the dishes are being done. Or a person could be a modernist of the dishes and make a stream of consciousness account of an attempt to flee dish-sink reality. But it would be easy for any of those accounts of doing the dishes to miss what is important about doing the dishes, which is that it is not interesting or remarkable work in itself, but that it is the work on which everything else depends.

An ongoing necessity like dirty dishes needing to be done doesn't produce narrative. It produces quantities, like how many dishes were washed. It produces temporal measurements, like how much time was spent washing them and when. Narratives end. Quantities, hours, and dishes don't.

Maybe dishes produce categories and distinctions. Maybe one kind of dish is washed but not the other, one kind of technique used and not another. To study the dishes could result in an account of spaces, of technologies, of tools and instruments, or infrastructures, economics. A work like that could demonstrate the crisis that occurs in its absence: the dishes have piled up, the smells and cockroaches have come. Or it could result in an account of class, race, and gender—who, in the current arrangement of the world, does the dishes and who does not.

Doing the dishes falls inside a larger set of relations made up of necessity. We have physical bodies. These exist inside and among the larger bodies of the world. All of these bodies—ours and everything else's—are adhered to decay, are always ruining or on the verge of it, never evade entropy or collapse. The ordinary ongoingness of our existence, like every time we do the dishes, is every time we try to block ruin's path.

There is the work of making the world, which is the world that's good to look at, and there is the quieter work of keeping the world okay once it is here. Making the world is a concrete pleasure, but the nature of the rest of it has yet to be determined. It's hard to make a judgment of the senses regarding the sometimes invisible and necessary efforts we exchange between us. It is hard to read, for beauty, the everywhere space we are always making around the always manifesting world of the world.

3.

It is usually someone's mother with cancer, at least in books, or their sister, or lover or wife. In literature, one person's cancer seems to exist as an instrument of another person's epiphanies, and sickness takes the form of how a sick person looks. At a poetry reading I attend during my illness, a poet is nearly shouting and wailing poems about a cancer she doesn't have, then another poet at another—everyone's mother—then a book comes in the mail in which the mother dying of cancer is, now that she is so thin and pale, compared with a long list of famous thin pale beauties. None of this literature is bad, but all of it is unforgivable.

Lepers were once called God's captives, an opportunity for charity, shouting "unclean, unclean" as they entered any city.[10] It is as if cancer patients shout "instrumentalize me, instrumentalize me" with only our looks.

I once had hair. I would brush it out and put it in a loose knot on top of my head, wash my face, pat on serums and lotions, wear pajamas, climb into a made bed, read myself to sleep, wake up in the morning and take down my hair, go to the bathroom and look in the mirror to see if anything about me had changed in the night. I would apply sunscreen, mascara, eyeliner, lipstick, earrings, check for chips in my nail polish, find pleasure in clothes and sex, feel hungry for food. Now I am ashamed that I had ever been so unphilosophical as to search in a mirror for a wrinkle, ashamed also about how I used to covet my physical pleasures in the manner of a miser whose tiny purse they believe to be full of riches but is full of nothing but carefully accounted-for decay. I am ashamed that I should ever have been like a dog who thought its purpose was in guarding the modest portion of deception and ephemerality that is sometimes mistaken for beauty. This is not anything I want anyone to know about me.

After one of my surgeries, I asked a friend to help me count my wounds. She said, "I don't like this," and looked like she was about to cry, like this was the sort of event that would end up in literature later, and I pleaded with her. I said "this is my body" and "I want to know what has happened to it" and "I was drugged and no one explained what they did to me" and "I don't even know how many holes I have."

I stood in front of the mirror with my compression garment pulled down past my waist. We looked at what we could see, one of us in horror, me in harsh, curious insistence. We couldn't figure out what were holes and what weren't, what the bruises meant, the blood spots, the abrasions. The pains in my body were not precise instructions for the future or reliable accounts of the past. The entire upper half hurt: *neck arms glands upper abdomen lower abdomen back eyeballs throat face shoulders head.* There was one spot, on the side of what would be my new left breast, that hurt like an emergency. There was one spot, on the side of what would be my new right breast, that hurt like a minor emergency.

What being a writer does to a person is make her a servant of those sensory details, obedient to the world of appearances and issuing forth book after book compliant with deceptive and unforgivable showing, full of cruel and unnecessary showing, irresponsibly sparing every ethically required telling, as telling is that other truth, and the senses are prone to showing's lies.

Showing is a betrayal of the real, which you can never quite know with your eyes in the first place, and if you are trying to survive for the purpose of literature, *showing and not telling* is not reason enough to endure the disabling processes required for staying alive.

The slightly ill but undiagnosed—the people who hover near hypochondriac—are better narrators. Their suffering is not so overdetermined. They can be lavishly self-defined, poetic with the glamour of the sick person's proximity to finality. They bear none of the weight of being specifically ill in specific body parts at a specific point in history with a specific and specifically gendered disease.

I do not want to tell the story of cancer in the way that I have been taught to tell it. The way I have been taught to tell the story is a person would be diagnosed, treated, either live or die. If she lives, she will be heroic. If she dies, she will be a plot point. If she lives, she will say something fierce, her fierceness applauded, or perform the absolutions of gratitude, her gratitude then praised. If she lives, she will be the angel of epiphany. If she dies, she will be the angel of epiphany. Or if she is allowed a voice, she can complain in fractured and enigmatic drips or corral situational cliché and/or made-for-TV sentimentality and/or patho-pornography into a good story. Literature sails along on every existing prejudice.

A single mother with breast cancer should be an opportunity for a sentimental projection worth a thousand country songs. She should be beautifully devised, donating her easy-to-see agony to the mythic accruals of art.

If this were a novel, a sick person would discover that she is a reincarnated version of Job, then find out that every other person alive is a reincarnated Job, too.

If this were sociology, experience would inhabit a set of categories. The sick person is, as they say, a deviant like all the other deviants. First, she will recognize that she is ill. Then her new role as *sick person* must be defined. The doctor fills out the paperwork for HR. If she is insured, the insurer is notified. If she isn't, and is poor enough, the social worker helps her fill out the Medicaid forms. The Facebook post is made, the head shaved in a photo-documented process of smiles and thumbs up. She begins to submit to treatments and to situate her disease progression in the social realm. She must appear to others as sick and begin to ask for help, establish her virtue in a plea for fund-raising and meal deliveries. People with cancer are not put in prisons or mental hospitals or homeless shelters like others who are considered deviant, although there are many sick people in all of those places, too, sick with cancer without a bed to sleep in or throwing up from chemotherapy inside a prison ward. But our hypothetical sick person, if cancer is her one big problem, rotates in and out of clinics and emergency rooms and intensive care, as if she is a car submitted for service that will keep it barely running but always coughing exhaust.

I would rather write nothing at all than propagandize for the world as is.

I am certain that my illness would make a better book if it were someone else's. Who would want to hear the hammer always complaining about its meeting with the nail? An object is an object for a reason. Or at least I tell myself this when the books others have written about people with cancer start to show up in the mail. These are always mailed with the best intentions, always about the sister, wife, or mother-in-law, all of the dying women with a bald head and none of them with a voice or much else to distinguish them in particular except they were surely once distinguishable people and by the time they made it into the books, weren't.

These books I am given read like proof that it should always be other people's faces that are swollen from steroids, not my own, not my own breasts gone now, replaced by glued skin and cold silicone. But I am, despite the literature, the sick one, the recipient of what seems to be all the dying-wife stories in the canon of cancer's accounts. Women's suffering is generalized into literary opportunity.

Cancer is in our time and place one of the most effective diseases at eradicating the precise and individual nature of anyone who has it, and feminized cancers—in that to be seen as a woman is also to be, in a way, semi-eradicated, this eradication deepened by class, race, and disability—even more so. Women with cancer are often forced to watch themselves dissolve, lamentable objects intolerable as lamenting ones, witnesses to everyone else's sad stories but socially corrected as soon as a sadness issues from their own mouths.

If you send me a literature in which a woman with cancer is herself, a complete, complex, and speaking person, I will open the mail. But what kept showing up was like the unrivaled suffering of some acquaintances with whom I'd often disagreed too much to call friends. They seemed to cry harder at my diagnosis than I did. All that unearned "so shook up" typed, overfamiliarly, toward me in chats by men who expected me to absorb their own excessive feeling on the occasion of my devastation.

A man I met once at a bar has decided to devote himself to my care, and his enthusiasm for my vulnerability is so great that I have to block his number from my phone. My friends and I sometimes joke about cancer chasers, or cancer daddies with CDs full of slow jams, the gifts showing up at the door, the outbreaks of attracted chivalry, the curious attempts at seduction. One friend suggests that whatever libidinal appeal cancer possesses has to do with the disease's nontransmissibility. Cancer's attraction is that it is a disease of probability rather than communicability, she tells me, and every person with cancer can be understood as someone who has cancer so you won't have to.

We share this world, the objects and environments in it, its systems, distribution, and manufacturing, the radioactive rays of the machines on which we seek to talk to one another, too, and all we know combines into the industrial world's carcinogenosphere. That we catch our disease from the shared world absolves us from fear of giving it to one another directly, and cancer allows proximity to the authentic experience without other diseases' proximate risks. Cancer can be a stage of virtue on which others can act, and it is also a pure instance of suffering in which we have no one—and everything—to blame.

Here is an exercise in lamentation without opportunism: walk down a street and imagine the unhappiness experienced behind every door, then, while moving through a town or city in a car or bus, observe every business and imagine what each of the workers would rather be doing than work. Then imagine those workers' parents, what they would rather be doing, too, or what they would rather the children that they raised could do.

The graveyard has the same effect. Each tombstone is like a Wikipedia stub unfilled.

Next, do the same thing, only this time, in front of a prison. Then do this in a hospital.

4.

I read somewhere that while many people have written histories of illness, no one has ever written a history of the ill. But I don't think this is true. Every person with a body is a secret historian, at work on the same volume: skin as the annals of sensation, genitals as jokes told by fools, teeth as the rise and fall of what bites.

I dream I am walking at three a.m. in the high streets of the suburbs which on a turn would become the low streets of the city, 140th Street to 18th Street, 196th to 3rd. These were the streets of every gridded place to which I had ever been, and I was worried because in the dream I had cancer and was weak, lost, and all around me in the streets and cars were celebrants before dawn. I knew that the celebrants were ordinary and, in this, dangerous to the sick in the way that celebrants almost always are.

Disease is never neutral. Treatment never not ideological. Mortality never without its politics.

Cancer is held apart as a special kind of suffering, but suffering from the inevitability of our common accident isn't valiant. To be a child of this accident never made me a member of a valiant class. Immobilized in bed, I decide to devote my life to making the socially acceptable response to news of a diagnosis of breast cancer not the corrective "stay positive," but these lines from Diane di Prima's poem "Revolutionary Letter #9": "1. kill head of Dow Chemical / 2. destroy plant / 3. MAKE IT UNPROF-ITABLE FOR THEM to build again."[11]

Moments of taking charge of ourselves foreground them-selves in a lot of forgettable necessity. An interesting story is made of agency, but humans exist as fully on this shadow side of helplessness as we do on the daylight side of doing what we want. To be cared for is the invisible sub-structure of autonomy, the necessary work brought about by the weakness of a human body across the span of life. Our gaze into the world is sometimes a needy one, a face that says "love me," by which it means something like "bring me some soup."

In infancy, this asking comes, in part, with a promised relationship to the future—love me, the face of a baby says, and it will be the cause of the future's beneficial ef-fect. Care for me, the helplessness of a baby says, so that I can be a person who will grow up and be able to care for others in turn.

When we are elderly, the face that says "love me" does so by evoking a remembered relationship to the past—love me, an elderly person's need says, and as the effect of the past's beneficial cause of the love I gave you or someone or something else.

But the unexpectedly sick person—the one incapacitated in their body when they should have, in the accepted social order, been doing something else, like caring for their own children or caring for the elderly around them or going to work—must cash in their *love me* from the collateral of every or any temporal experience, calling in the past, playing on hopes for the future.

Love me, the sick person in the prime of their life says, trying to look as if they will grow strong again, for what I have done before, and also what I might do, and also love me for the present in which I am eternally trapped, uncertain of my exact attachment to time.

The title of the past four days has been *Neutropenia in the Time of Enterovirus*. My blood counts show that my immune system barely exists. I have been unable to be around people, afraid of becoming deathly ill, not just from the enterovirus but threats like the common cold or invisible mold on refrigerated food. My friend Cara has taken away all my houseplants for fear I might become sick from the soil's microbes. When people bring me flowers, she takes these, too. The only time I leave my apartment is to take walks alone. On one of these walks I forgot myself, petted a large black poodle, then remained in fear of my own hands for a mile.

In Goethe's *Faust*, Mephistopheles takes the form of a black poodle, follows at Faust's heels. When others see the poodle, they see only a dog, but when Faust sees it, he sees future fetters being woven around his feet. The poodle growls, and Faust tells it to be quiet.[12] I read somewhere that when Faust says, "Be quiet, poodle!" he is actually speaking to himself.[13]

Every day then, as I still do now, I swear that I will never again reproduce the battered account that happened in my notebook the day before.

I have always hated every shade of the heroic, but that doesn't mean I've never had that look. The common struggle gets pushed through the sieve of what forms we have to make its account, and before you know it, the wide and shared suffering of this world is narrowed and gossamer, as thin as silk and looking as special as the language it takes to tell it.

Language is common, too, but in the same insidious processes of finding a way to tell, language gets attached as property to its teller, as if the singularity of any given mouth is a singularity of having been born, or having felt pain, having been scared or having needed care, having set out to interpret the uninterpretable dream of waking up each day to the worst. The telling is always trying to slide down into a reinforcement of the conditions that made us want to say something in the first place, rather than their exposé, as if the gravity of our shared diminishments is more powerful than any ascendant rage.

Keenly felt suffering gets assigned to one type—some elegant specialist's languorous and pale upper-class faintness of being—and in its telling, comes out looking, no matter the reality, like a treasure of that class.

If you didn't know me, you might think, too, that my illness was so precious it was merely a suffering for the sake of semiotics, that I sat in the infusion room thinking only of Ancient Rome. But I was a single mother without savings who existed in a world of profit, had no partner to care for me or family nearby in a world that privatizes survival, had to work all through my treatment at a job where I was advised to never let on I was ill, had never had wealth or been proximate to the seats of power. In other words, my cancer, like almost anyone else's, was ordinary, as was, apart from my practice of writing, my life.

My cancer was not just a set of sensations nor lessons in interpretation nor a problem for art, although it was all of these things, too. My cancer was a captive fear that I would die and leave my daughter in a hard world with no resources, a fear, too, that I had devoted my life to writing and sacrificed all I had to never come to its reward. It was a terror that all I'd ever written would sit data-mined but not read in Google's servers until even Google's servers were made of dust, and in the meantime, I would become that unspeaking thing, a dead person, leaving too soon who and what I loved the most behind, unprotected, and alone.

The deer struggled to get up, then fell, then struggled to its feet, slumped its way into the bank parking lot after being hit by a car. My daughter, who was fourteen years old at the time, said,

"Anne, I hate what the world has done to the world."

and

"The only choice left is terrorist or shut-in."

I tell my daughter that my BRCA genetic test came back negative. I tell her that without a hormonal cause and without a genetic tendency and without obvious lifestyle factors the cancer I had probably just came from exposure to radiation or random carcinogens, that she doesn't have to worry that she is predisposed or genetically cursed.

"You forget," she answered, "that I still have the curse of living in the world that made you sick."

Every person with a body should be given a guide to dying as soon as they are born.

5.

A problem with art as it approaches suffering is that those who suffer are so often worn out from having suffered that any account of that suffering is exhausted before it is even tried. I was tired, and up against the problem of needing to tell what happened in the presence, too, of vulnerability's difficult sublimity and everything else rumored to be ineffable. How could I write about the world as it is when it is the same world that was guilty of this body (mine), which in all of its senses felt only like the animate form of its own betrayal?

It sometimes feels more painful to talk about having cancer than to have it. It feels more difficult to re-create the experience and impressions of an illness than to endure them. It is more trying to look into the scene from the center of the scene, to contort like that toward the true, than to turn one's head and lower one's eyes and get through as others have gotten through, accepting what's told to them, hoping for the mercies of forgetting.

I would prefer to write about anything else. "But the truth," wrote Bertolt Brecht, in an essay about the difficulties involved with writing it, "cannot merely be written; it must be written for someone, someone who can do something with it."[14] I would rather write about anything else, not only for fear of the pain of examining the pain, but also for fear of turning the pain into a product. I would rather write about anything else, not just for fear of telling the same story, but for fear that the "same story" is a lie in service of the way things are. I would rather write about anything else, but I know that other people exist, all of us with bodies inside history, all of us with nervous systems and nightmares, all of us with environments and hours and desires, like the one to not be sick, or to not get sick, or to understand what it means when we are.

A writer must, wrote Brecht, be courageous enough to know the truth, keen enough to recognize it, skillful enough to weaponize it, judicious enough to know who might be able to use it, and cunning enough to help it find its way.[15] And the truth must be written for someone, a someone who is all of us, all who exist in that push and pull of what bonds of love tie us to the earth and what suffering drives us from it.

Back in the Roman Empire, Aelius Aristides had a problem. He wanted to write a book, but he didn't know how to organize the information of his experience:

> Since I have mentioned the river and the terrible winter and the bath, am I next to speak of other things of the same category and am I to compile, as it were, a catalogue of wintry, divine, and very strange baths? Or dividing up my tale, shall I narrate some intermediate events? Or is it best to pass over all the intermediate things and give an end to my first tale, how the oracle about the years held and how everything turned out?[16]

__ HOW THE ORACLE HELD

-
-
-
—
-
-
-
—
-
-
-
—
-
-
-
—
-
-
-

1.

After the cancer has you, you forget how much life you have lost to living, and also how much of yourself you have lost to illness because it is difficult to take care of the illness and to take care of yourself as well. To take care of your illness can become the whole reason for existing, a marriage arranged by fate, and later when it isn't the acute illness stealing life from life it is the chronic disabling conditions left over from curing it, too.

Cancer then feels quaintly catastrophic in the manner of the previous century, the one from which my cancer's treatments are carried over, as are its causes. It is as if I am both sick with and treated by the twentieth century, its weapons and pesticides, its epic generalizations and its expensive festivals of death. Then, sick beyond sick from that century, I am made sick, again, from information—a sickness that is our century's own.

In the industrialized world, an estimated half of us have cancer, or will get it, and most everyone, even if we don't know it, is carrying a little bit of it around. Cancer doesn't even really exist, at least not as itself. Cancer is an idea we cast as an aspersion over our own malignancy.

That we carry around errant cells in breasts and prostates and lungs is not the crisis. Cancer becomes a crisis twice: once, upon its discovery, and next, in its discovery's effect. Its effect is most often a calamity of medicine, or a calamity of its absence, the first orchestrated in prevention of the calamity of death, which, along with birth, is the least unique calamity on earth.

Under the conditions of these calamities, there is no listening to my body, which in these circumstances keeps saying the wrong things. My body feels like it is dying as a side effect of what is promised to keep it alive, and requests, as its preservation, its destruction: to not move, to not eat, to not work, to not sleep, to refuse all touch. Every nerve is a beggar, asking for the alms of an end. Any wisdom of my body comes out as an insufferably melodramatic request made by a fool. I had to believe, however, that all my body meant by wanting to die then was not that it hated life, only that it could no longer bear this.

Then my body bore the unbearable, as many of ours do. Sometimes the only way to survive the worst is to run to the perfect refuge of being dulled. Disassociation reigns, but no one minds your daydreaming when you are sick with cancer. Some friends appear to wish that I would disassociate more, that I would give up my love of lucidity through events better survived in mental retreat.

Despite icing my hands and feet all during chemotherapy in an attempt to avoid it, my fingernails and toenails begin to lift from their beds. Fingernails lifting from fingers hurt as badly as fingernails lifting from fingers should. I bandage my iridescently painted nails onto me. I've lost friends, lovers, memory, eyelashes, and money to this illness, so I am stubbornly opposed to losing anything else to which I am attached. My nails fall off despite my opposition.

My nerves begin to die, disintegrating into a sizzling sensation from their ends in my fingers, toes, and genitals. Then my fingers are the most annoying solipsists: numb to the world, outraged in their interiors. *Your Oncology*

Journey says the solution to this condition, neuropathy, is to ask others to button my shirt, but it doesn't explain who. I'm made clumsy by altered proprioception, too. I can no longer trust my feet to tell me where I stand.

A woman I know tells me that she, as she had once known herself, has never really returned from the cancer she had thirty years ago. Now in her seventies, she says that she goes to work and comes home each day to spend her hours in disassociated blankness, and because she has to work for a living, must go there once more in the morning and pretend that she exists again. Some of us who survive the worst survive it into bare inexistence. Aelius Aristides described this, too: "Thus I was conscious of myself as if I were another person, and I perceived my body ever slipping away, until I was nearly dead."

I think of the medieval Islamic philosopher Avicenna's floating man, who, denied all sensation, still knows, as proof of the soul, that he exists.[1] I am not sure I believe him. A better answer is found in the Roman poet Lucretius's argument in his epic poem, *De rerum natura*, that we can die inch by inch. Every cell is a kingdom of both substance and spirit, and any kingdom can be overthrown. Our life force, like our flesh, never seems to issue away from us all at once. Anyone who has been half dead can attest to this. What we call our soul can die in small quantities, just as our bodies can be worn, amputated, and poisoned away, bit by bit.[2] The lost parts of our souls are no more replaceable than the lost parts of our bodies, life incrementally lifting from life, just like that. And there we are, mostly dead, but still required to go to work.

All that's left from before is the vague term "myself," which I now can compare with cancer's impersonal irreality. For a long time once it all gets going, I feel as if I am probably dead, haunting the earth's slightly familiar territory, a postbiological traveler to an afterlife in which for whatever reason I am sometimes allowed to believe that I am alive and achieving modest success. If I were still alive, I thought, I'd have at least visited California. If this were really life, I thought, there's no way that many people would have read my book of poetry. If I am dead, I am at least pleased that the administrators of eternity have assigned me a morally complex and moderately pleasurable afterworld.

It is awkward, over dinner, when I admit to people that I might not be alive. There is, too, a difficulty in trying to prove to yourself that you exist. It would take a newsfeed the duration of the cosmos to remind you of what you actually are, the constant insistent scrolling of that proof, the friends you once had, the mistakes you made, the feelings you hurt, all the beds you slept in, all the books you read, the enemies who consider you now too pitiable to be a rival, the way you looked in those days versus the way you now appear. Memory is that newsfeed for those who have been allowed to keep their minds intact, but I am not so lucky, having had to exchange mine for my life. Real literature would be *Proust in Bed*, about an affluent man who is deeply interested in his mother. My book should be called *The Medically Induced Failure of the Remembrance of Things Past*.

I read later that feeling like you are dead can have its mechanical cause in certain kinds of brain damage, such as the kind I've endured from chemotherapy. I'm a ghost, but my loss of me isn't even metaphysical—it's mechanical. Yet the rational explanation of why I feel dead half the time does little to mediate the irrational horror of existing in a way that I feel I don't exist. Here we are, here I am, alone and myself, half of me fallen off, half of us gone, and all of us as ghosts or the undying ones, half of us dead and half of myself nowhere to be remembered or to be found.

2.

In 1974, the year the FDA approved the chemo drug Adria-mycin, the British novelist D. G. Compton published *The Continuous Katherine Mortenhoe*, a novel about, among other things, a woman who has been told that she is about to die. Mortenhoe is diagnosed with a fatal case of Gordon's syndrome, a disease half caused by in-formation overload, the "inherent physical limits to the amounts and speeds of image processing possible in the human brain."[3] But a person with Gordon's syndrome isn't only dying of information: she is dying of her out-raged response to it. What Mortenhoe is told she is dying of is the kind of outrage that comes after a person has been inundated with data, screen after screen of it. It's a perpetual state of outrage over information that has caused Mortenhoe's mind, her doctor explains, to fatally resist the structures of the world, creating, as he says, "a pattern of rebellion."[4] He says nothing can be done— she's been too sick and too relentlessly oppositional. A computer has measured out the rest of her life for her: she has a month to live. Katherine Mortenhoe has to die because in response to the world and all the information in it, her brain is in the constant state of wanting to throw up.

Mortenhoe works at a publishing house called Computabook. As she waits for news of her illness, she enters plots into a computer program, named Barbara, that writes novels. Upon finding out that she herself is dying of "burned out circuits," Mortenhoe begins to pity the computer program she works with, whose circuits are also overworked—"Poor Barbara," she repeats. Mortenhoe begins to imagine a literature written in the old-fashioned way, without the intervention of the machines. She would write a book that would include people as they really are, she thinks, "each one simply chemistry, simply a bundle of neurons, each bundle equipped with an internal communications system built up down life's millennia for reasons mostly obsolete."[5]

Mortenhoe works in the Romance division—she *is* the Romance division, Romance's sole manager and employee—so it is no surprise that despite her cybernetic positivism she goes on to think, "My story will contain the only reality, that there is no reality, and it will make me famous. I shall write it possibly in the hospital, possibly dictating the last chapters as I die."[6]

Mortenhoe is dying of disease in a world where almost everyone now dies of old age, and for this reason, she becomes a minor celebrity. To satisfy a "pain-starved public," the media has begun to follow her, hoping for photo opportunities. To keep them at bay, Mortenhoe fills out the paperwork to get a permit for three days of "private grief."

In the capitalist medical universe in which all bodies must orbit around profit at all times, even a double mastectomy is considered an outpatient procedure. After my mastectomy, the eviction from the recovery ward came aggressively and early. The nurse woke me up from anesthesia and attempted to incorrectly fill out all the questions on the exit questionnaire for me while I failed in an attempt to argue with her that I was not okay. I told her that my pain was not managed, that I had not yet actually gone to the bathroom, that I had not yet been given instructions, that I could not stand, let alone leave. Then they made me leave, and I left.

You can't drive yourself home the same day you have had a double mastectomy, of course, whimpering in pain, unable to use your arms, with four drainage bags hanging from your torso, delirious from anesthesia and barely able to walk. You are not supposed to be alone when you get home, either. But no one really asks how you manage it once you are forced out of the surgical center—who, if anyone, you have to care for you, what sacrifices these caregivers might have to make or the support they require.

It should be no surprise that single women with breast cancer, even adjusting for age, race, and income, die of it at up to twice the rate of the married. The death rate gets higher if you are single and poor.

Everyone understands as a matter of fact that unless you are currently entered into this world's customary romantic partnership, or unless you have lived long enough to raise devoted grown children, or unless you are young enough to still be in the care of your parents, you are, on the occasion of aggressive cancer in the conditions of aggressive profit, rarely considered worth enough to keep alive.

When Fanny Burney underwent an unanesthetized mastectomy in her Paris bedroom in September 1811 for the lump she discovered the previous August, one of her doctors told her, "il faut s'attendre à souffrir. Je ne veux pas vous tromper—Vous souffrirez—vous souffrirez *beaucoup*!"

You, the surgeon told her, *will suffer a lot*.

Burney wrote of her tumor, "I felt the evil to be deep, so deep that I often thought if it could not be dissolved, it could only with life be extirpated." Weighing a long, painful death by cancer against a short, painful death by its potential cure, she submitted herself to the most optimistic form of suffering. She elected to have the tumor removed.

Seven surgeons arrived in dark robes. Climbing into the makeshift surgical bed and lying with a veil over her eyes, Burney hears the lead surgeon ask, "Qui me tiendra ce sein?" ("Who will hold this breast for me?"), to which she replies, "I will, sir." She rips off her veil, cradles her own breast in her hand so that the surgeon can begin to amputate it, and explains in detail its radiant web of pain.

At that, the surgeon quietly replaces the veil and puts Burney's hand back by her side. "Hopeless, then," she writes, "desperate, and self-given up, I closed once more my Eyes, relinquishing all watching, all resistance, all interference, and sadly resolute to be wholly resigned."

"They felt as if hermetically shut," wrote Burney of her eyes during the surgery.[7]

Suffering doesn't need to be witnessed to be experienced, and in the case of illness, loss remains, as a source of knowledge, supreme. As in that other famous literary account of a mastectomy—Audre Lorde's, in which she is anesthetized; then, as she describes in *The Cancer Journals*, wakes up biopsied, terrified, and transformed—a person's full participation in loss is also to make an account of how, by necessity of experience, one's full participation is foreclosed. To have a body means you will not always see what has happened to it.

In Burney's case, to see what was happening would have been unbearable. Even with her eyes shut, she passed out twice. In order to keep knowing, she relinquished all watching. The account she gives is that which steps beyond the testimony of any eye, which is a testimony to illness's something else, that realm of experience beyond the visual. On March 25, 1978, Audre Lorde wrote:

> The idea of knowing, rather than believing, trusting, or even understanding, has always been considered heretical. But I would willingly pay whatever price in pain was needed, to savor the weight of contemplation; to be utterly filled, not with conviction nor with faith, but with experience—knowledge, direct and different from all other certainties.[8]

Knowing is something other—for anyone but the expert class, accusable and doubted. And as feeling forbids watching, strong feeling can also impede thinking, or at least in the case of Burney, who writes that her feelings about the event of her mastectomy make her unable to think of the event. But to not be able to think doesn't mean to not know. Even nine months after her mastectomy, and in the three months it takes to write an account of it down, Burney writes that she can't reread what she has written without feeling sick. What she has written is not simply an account of a mastectomy. It is an account of that which we must witness but which we cannot allow our eyes to see, of that which we must understand but cannot stand to think about, and of that which we know we must write down but find unbearable to read.

To think about this makes me sick, and to write about it, too, and to read the accounts of the mastectomies of others is often also unbearable. I feel sick, too, about how I am sometimes envious of the horrible circumstances of the past because they are at least differently horrible and differently degraded than our era's own.

In the 1970s, Audre Lorde, according to *The Cancer Journals*, spent five days in the hospital being cared for after the removal of one of her breasts.[9] Lorde had a hospital room in which she could have visitors, a bed to rest in, was able to start walking through the halls before she walked into her home again, was able to spend weeks recovering, too, and to think of the loss of her breast— not the loss of her capacity to remember, use words, and to think as a result of chemotherapy—as her cancer's primary event. Despite the lie of progress, so many people with breast cancer don't get any of this anymore, nor adequate pain control on leaving surgery, nor physical therapy for postmastectomy pain and mobility issues, nor time off work, nor is the loss of a breast nearly their biggest postcancer problem. While they don't get a hospital bed to recover in or rehabilitation for the cognitive damage incurred during their treatment, what they do get in the United States is federally mandated access to breast reconstruction—any type of implant they want.

When reading historical accounts of breast cancer, I am often struck by a world on which profit hadn't taken such a full and festering hold. Now, despite inadequate advancement in postsurgical pain management, a patient's breasts are often cut off, tissue banked and incinerated, then the patient is forced onto her feet and out of bed. What I and so many others experience now are called "drive-by mastectomies." According to one study by the federal Agency for Healthcare Research and Quality, "45 percent of mastectomies in 2013 were performed in hospital-affiliated outpatient surgery centers with no overnight stay."[10] No matter how eloquently we argue from our recovery beds that we need care after we've been cut open, when we are bleeding, raw, shocked, agonized, and drugged, we are not allowed it.

I have to go back to work ten days after a double mastectomy and the beginning of chest expander reconstruction. I've been teaching all through the months of chemotherapy before my surgery, but despite this, I've run out of medical leave. I would have given up access to every silicone implant in the world to be guaranteed that the career I had built would be still around for me if I could take some time off to treat my cancer, but if one's cancer treatment exceeds that narrow window of the FMLA's weeks of unpaid leave, there can be no guarantee.

I'm angry about how much I require myself inside these conditions to refuse to admit the pain that Lorde and Burney and the others before me have so expertly described. I attempt not to feel anything about my mastectomy because to feel the full weight of these events—particularly after half a year of aggressive chemotherapy—would eviscerate the last of my capacity to survive them. I do not mourn my own lost breasts, because the condition of the shared world seems exponentially more grievable.

I'm angry that days after surgery I have little choice but to be driven to work by my friends, all of whom have already had to make great sacrifices to help me, who must carry my books into the classroom for me because I can't use my arms. Delirious from pain and loss in those days after my surgery, I give a three-hour lecture on Walt Whitman's poem "The Sleepers"—"wandering and confused, lost to myself, ill-assorted, contradictory"—with surgical drainage bags stitched to my tightly compressed chest, expected to be bravely visible as a breast cancer survivor while my students have no idea what has been done to me or how much I hurt.

A person who complains about any aspect of breast cancer treatment in public is often drowned out by a chorus
of people, many of whom have never had cancer, accus-
ing her of ingratitude, saying she is lucky, warning her
that her bad attitude might kill her, reminding her she
could be dead. Like anyone else with cancer, I am told to
be grateful—that I have access to treatment, that I have a
meaningful job, that I have friends, that I have, thus far,
lived—because it will ease my recovery, and I really am,
I guess. As Whitman wrote in "The Sleepers": "Whoever
is not in his coffin and the dark grave, let him know he
has enough." My permit for private grief has long ex-
pired like everyone else's.

It's probably obvious now that many aspects of experience are so visible and yet many conditions are worse, such struggled-for awareness mostly a disappointing variable of acquiescence, struggled for again and again, only to disappoint again as newly ordinary. Visibility doesn't reliably change the relations of power to who or what is visible except insofar as visible prey are easier to hunt.

People die visibly, worry visibly, suffer visibly, the whole world opened up to the surveillance of the whole world. The drone pilots kill their visible victims. The corporations data-mine our visible correspondence and count our visible clicks. We post our agonies in our visible support groups. The satellite skies look down on our visible everything although the birds and clouds remain blissfully indifferent, and on the medical screens, once-private interiors are now visible, inside out. Most everyone alive now is smart enough to know that there is an ominous visibility to all that was once directly lived. Identifying a problem brings little of the resolution we really want to it, only now we have the extra work of signal-boosting the

common tragedy inside its corporate structure of delim-
ited truth.

And in the tragedy of the tragedy, and in my contradictions, which I suspect aren't too different from all of yours,
this doesn't mean there aren't so many sad and wrong and
outrageous things I want everyone to know. Some things,
however, remain mysterious and unspectacular, and in
this, I think, there is hope. The fate of the world relies on
the promise of the negative, just as we can rely that sight
is not the only sense.

3.

I have always wanted to write the most beautiful book against beauty. I'd call it *Cyclophosphamide, doxorubicin, paclitaxel, docetaxel, carboplatin, steroids, anti-inflammatories, antipsychotic antinausea meds, anti-anxiety antinausea meds, antinausea meds, antidepressants, sedatives, saline flushes, acid reducers, eyedrops, eardrops, numbing creams, alcohol wipes, blood thinners, antihistamines, antibiotics, antifungals, antibacterials, sleep aids, D_3, B_{12}, B_6, joints and oils and edibles, hydrocodone, oxycodone, fentanyl, morphine, eyebrow pencils, face creams.*

Then the surgeon called to tell me that as far as she could tell, the drugs had worked, the cancer is gone. The double mastectomy performed after six months of chemotherapy revealed a "pathologic complete response," the outcome I'd hoped for, the one that gave me the greatest chance that when I die, it won't be of this.

With that news, I am like a baby being born into the hands of a body made only of the grand debt of love and rage, and if I live another forty-one years to avenge what has happened it still won't be enough.

_ THE HOAX

If Heaven I cannot bend, then Hell I will arouse.

—Epigraph to Freud's *Interpretation of Dreams*, 1899

1.

I come across a headline: "Attitude Is Everything for Breast Cancer Survivor." I look for the headline "Attitude Is Everything for Ebola Patient" or "Attitude Is Everything for Guy with Diabetes" or "Attitude Is Everything for Those with Congenital Syphilis" or "Attitude Is Everything with Lead Poisoning" or "Attitude Is Everything When a Dog Bites Your Hand" or "Attitude Is Everything for Gunshot Victim" or "Attitude Is Everything for a Tween with a Hangover" or "Attitude Is Everything for a Coyote Struck by a Ford F150" or "Attitude Is Everything for Gravity" or "Attitude Is Everything for the Water Cycle" or "Attitude Is Everything for Survivor of Varicose Veins" or "Attitude Is Everything for Dying Coral Reef."

2.

After the kids at the school he worked at raised funds for him, an Oklahoma teacher's aide named Ken MaBone was given the keys to a new car to drive himself to cancer treatment.[1] The friends of Jenifer Gaskin, a single mother in Oregon, arranged a meal rotation for the duration of her treatment so that she and her children would have something to eat.[2] Alicia Pierini tattooed this phrase on her upper arm in italics: "Cancer may have started the fight but I will finish it."[3]

The chemotherapy regime Maggie endured made it difficult to walk. Monica broke her leg in two places after her first chemotherapy infusion. Robert lost almost all of his teeth from chemotherapy and began to twitch uncontrollably. John Ingram endured chronic pain from the removal of breast tissue. Diane Green said about the consequence of her mastectomy: "I lost my home, I lost my marriage, I lost my health, I lost my job, I lost absolutely everything."[4]

In 2014, Belle Gibson, an Australian lifestyle blogger and author of *The Whole Pantry*, was declared by *ELLE* magazine "the most inspiring woman you've met this year." Belle, who claimed to be treating her cancer with diet, said she had cancer of the blood, spleen, brain, uterus, and liver. Except that she didn't.[5]

According to published reports, none of these people had cancer. Not the ones who were given cars or the ones who got tattoos or the ones who were given chemotherapy or the ones who endured surgery or the ones who wrote books. Some, like John Ingram and Diane Green, were led to believe by their doctors that they had cancer when they didn't. Others, like Ken MaBone, Jenifer Gaskin, Alicia Pierini, and Belle Gibson, allegedly led others to believe they had cancer when the evidence suggests that they themselves knew this was not true.

Farid Fata, an oncologist in Michigan, was sentenced to forty-five years in prison for administering chemotherapy to people without cancer.[6] The U.K. breast surgeon Ian Paterson was sentenced to fifteen years for removing people's breasts after leading his patients to believe that harmless conditions were malignant. "I have to pay for my holidays somehow," he is said to have joked before he was finally convicted of "wounding with intent."[7]

Some people are lied to about having cancer. Some people lie about having it. The world is full of anecdotal accounts of cancer fakers, all of whom seem to just want what everyone needs and deserves, some time off, a little spending money, a casserole in the fridge, some love. There are the stories like the one of the man who took a hundred days off from work with forged notes, or the woman who shaved her head and asked for donations at church, or the sister who turned her HPV into full-on cervical cancer for leverage at the holiday dinner table. There are also the doctors who mislead people with benign or mild cancer-related conditions into aggressive, expensive treatment, or the doctors who do not tell patients they are dying, leading them into months of costly, painful, useless interventions. The people who fake having cancer, when found out, often face, if not legal prosecution, social ostracism. The doctors who subtly overtreat patients often don't.

It isn't only doctors and patients who do the lying. The researcher Roger Poisson admitted to fabricating or falsifying treatment study data on almost a hundred patients involved in a landmark breast cancer study between the years 1977 and 1990. Poisson claims he tampered with the records for the good of his research subjects, many of whom he included in his studies despite their ineligibility. According to a *TIME* magazine article called "Great Science Frauds," "investigators found two sets of patient books in Poisson's lab, one marked 'true' and another labelled 'false.'"[8]

In September 2017, a large multidistrict litigation was filed stating that the manufacturer Sanofi-Aventis failed to adequately warn patients and doctors about life-altering adverse side effects of Taxotere. As early as 2009, the FDA had sent warning letters to Sanofi that some of its claims about the drug were false.[9] In another case, in July 2017, the pharmaceutical manufacturer Celgene agreed to pay $280 million in claims that it marketed cancer drugs for unapproved uses.[10] Increasingly, claims the FDA, "bogus remedies claiming to cure cancer in cats and dogs are showing up online."[11]

According to news reports, a British woman, Kelsey Whitehead, thirty-eight, shaved off her hair, used makeup to create the effect of illness, and forced herself to vomit at work. She bought a Hickman line—a surgically implanted port sometimes used for the administration of chemotherapy—and cut open her own chest to insert it. The judge who sentenced her for fraud told her she had "a real psychological problem."[12]

The pharmaceutical companies lie. The doctors lie. The sick lie. The healthy lie. The researchers lie. The Internet lies.

Cureyourowncancer.org, which sells cannabis oils and $45 snapback hats with a hemp leaf logo and the phrase "I kill cancer," claims, "Big Pharma lies to convince us that their so-called cancer 'cures' work." The description under the nine-minute-and-forty-four-second YouTube video "The Cancer Hoax Explained" simply reads: "The Medical Industry Kills You."

Every month is Pinktober when you have breast cancer, and every actual October is a season in hell. The world is blood pink with respectability politics, as if anyone who dies from breast cancer has died of a bad attitude or eating a sausage or not trusting the word of a junior oncologist. After my chemotherapy seems to work, people say how they knew that I, of course, would survive, as if I were someone so special and strong and all the others weren't.

Online forums keep ongoing accounts of losses from breast cancer. The women post stories about themselves as contented survivors walking into the doctor's office to treat a headache and then learning that they are dying of aggressive metastatic cancer, an answer to a question they never asked. The women say goodbye to the Facebook groups, email lists, and forums, or their partners do. The women know when they will die, which is too soon. Some will do anything to live, and then they die of that.

These are not the deserving dead. The pink ribbon cop cars and pink handcuffs and pink spirit-wear and pink ping-pong balls and pink plastic water bottles and pink revolvers should not be mistaken for a progress that the dying women somehow disappoint. Pink ribbons adorn the objects and processes that kill people. There is no cure and never has been.

In the United States, more than forty thousand people die of breast cancer each year: that's one woman dying of breast cancer about every thirteen minutes. If chemotherapy is too late or the wrong kind or otherwise ineffective, triple negative—the type of breast cancer I have—leaves the breast quickly, gallops over the body, and blooms in the body's soft parts: brain, lungs, liver. Then you can't breathe, can't live, can't think.

Many people, of course, don't know that there are *breast cancers*, plural, or the difference between one kind and another, or that anyone with breast tissue can get breast cancer, men and women and nonbinary people, cis and trans, young and old, fit and infirm, straight and queer. No cancer is a good cancer, but the people with the more common, hormone-receptor-positive breast cancers can often take tamoxifen, eat soy, look to the future, say in the cancer chat rooms, as they did so often that I couldn't bring myself to look, "at least I am not triple negative." And although most people with Stage 4 breast cancer will probably die of it, those with hormone-receptor-positive breast cancers know that if their cancer metastasizes, there is a chance it could do this slowly, choosing as its first site of invasion the slow hard substance of their bones, allowing them some time to live.

The women in online groups who are in the fourth stage of triple-negative cancer aren't likely to think in years. They post about their basal-type cells replicating fast, of the glowing spots on their brains. Others post of their fears of the feeling of dizziness or a cold that won't go away or is-it-cognitive-damage-left-over-from-chemo-or-is-it-a-tumor-in-my-brain or being at work with nerve-dead hands that can't manage a keyboard or hold a pen. Triple negative strikes black women disproportionately, and because of medicine's institutionalized racism, I think, has been the last breast cancer left with no targeted treatment. It also disproportionately afflicts the young, is a cancer that appears to operate with the logic that the healthier the body, the more aggressive and deadly it will be. "The good news," the oncologist said when he first introduced me to our pathology, "is that at least there is chemo." These women's deaths are racist and unnecessary, and our grief over them should tear open the earth.

The women on the forums who live call the women who have died "angels." Some women's lives follow closely another set of grim statistics: during active treatment, but particularly after it, they are abandoned, divorced, cheated on, abused, disabled, fired. Poverty and heartbreak both take iatrogenic forms: it is medical treatment, not the disease, that seems to cause them. On social media, the accounts of dying of a disease so many people mistake for curable weave into the accounts of breast cancer survivors being abandoned and impoverished, unemployable and brain-damaged and in pain. These weave into the posts, too, of my friends and acquaintances, their political debates and literary scandals and well-informed opinions, and weave, too, into news of police shootings, climate despair, action on the streets.

On an email list I joined the summer after treatment, patients from all over the world commiserated about living with the grievous effects of one of our chemotherapy drugs. We wrote to one another about the triumph of persuading the FDA to issue warnings about the drug, and once the legal battles started, over whether or not the drug company misrepresented its efforts. We made jokes about the ambulance-chasing commercials on national TV. "The most blatant case of failure to disclose in the history of the pharmaceutical industry" is what the lawyer I could never bring myself to hire for a lawsuit I didn't have the energy to pursue said to me. In the months after my treatment when I learned that I, too, would suffer for the rest of my life from the previously undisclosed side effects of this drug, I was unable to stomach devoting my survival to a lawsuit. By the time I could bring myself to call to get the records to confirm which lot of the drug I was given, the lawsuits had become public and my records couldn't be tracked down. I'll never know if these two facts are related. Years later, despite not joining the suit, I learned that the lawyers for the drug company had subpoenaed my email data for merely participating in the support group. I had to find a lawyer in order to try to stop my story from becoming part of a lawsuit against my will, and although I didn't want cancer, or the drug, or the lifelong consequences of the drug, or to participate in the lawsuit about the alleged lifelong consequences of the drug, it began to feel as if the aftermath of the aftermath of cancer treatment might never end. A nonprofit dedicated to consumer privacy helped me, but I still feel like the drug company that did this will—like cancer itself—always be looming, waiting to knock at my door.

Too many women I know say they wish they had chosen, instead of treatment by drugs with mutilating and disabling effects, to die of their cancer. The ever-after of our profit-and-drug-damaged lives has been too much for them to bear. But this is a false dilemma. In the case of the drug in question, it looks like there were other drugs available that were just as effective with less risk of permanent harm, but the drug we were treated with and that hurt us was, to someone, seemingly the more profitable choice. Some women send suicide notes, too, saying they can't go on living. These emails weave into my other emails, the ones from work and Ulta and editors, an eviscerating sadness sailing across information's level plane.

You will understand, I hope, that because of all of this, every pink ribbon looks like the flag of a conqueror stuck in a woman's grave.

3.

In a video entitled "I'm Dead =(" the vlogger Coopdizzle,
a self-described mother and wife who recorded the video
in her last days of life with triple-negative breast cancer,
said, "When you get cancer it is such an eye opener." I first
learn about Coopdizzle because she has left a comment
under the video of another triple-negative breast cancer
patient, Christina Newman, whose videos I begin to
watch after I am diagnosed.

In a 2011 video, "Why I Rejected Chemo & Radiation,"
Christina Newman describes how she decided to try to
heal her cancer with diet. Coopdizzle comments under
that particular video that it is Christina Newman's story
that has inspired her to go along with standard medical
treatment. After this comment, I begin to follow Coopdizzle's videos, too, because Christina Newman's story
had the same effect on me. It's because of Christina that I
keep going to chemotherapy even when I don't want to.
Following an unsuccessful attempt to treat her cancer
with diet, Christina Newman eventually turns to chemotherapy and warns others away from her earlier choices.

The diagnosis of Newman's spreading cancer came to her in a set of increasingly painful revelations. Christina says that she began to feel off, and despite her insistence that something was wrong, she said the doctors dismissed her concerns as posttreatment complaints and missed that she was pregnant. She gave birth to a daughter, Ava, in a surprise birth during a dangerous episode of preeclampsia. With her symptoms still not resolved, Christina kept complaining to doctors, who she said continued to push aside her concerns, now dismissing her complaints as postnatal. According to Newman, they said that they doubted they would find anything until they did find something. What they eventually found was that her liver was full of aggressive triple-negative cancer and that she was dying, a new infant in her care. Under the video in which Christina Newman announced her first decision to reject chemotherapy—the first scene of a story that turns into that cascading nightmare—someone has written, "To all you herbalists and natural alternative medicine bullshit con artists, THIS is what happens when you spew your bullshit."

In the video entitled "Final DAILY family vlog. The news is getting worse #72," Christina's partner says, "She's not ready to give up. She don't want to give up." It's Christina's last post. I remember first watching this video in the early weeks of my cancer treatment, grief-stricken for

Christina and terrified for myself. Christina was still alive then, sitting next to her partner, breathing oxygen through a tube, barely able to talk, her face rounded by steroids. It's the last I and her other viewers ever saw of her. The videos that follow it are from a friend who describes Christina's last hours alive, how much she wanted to record more YouTube videos, the way she seemed upset as the priest administered the last rites, the difficult hours after that it took for her to die.

On Christina's YouTube page someone congratulates Christina, no longer living, on her number of followers. A commenter named Tommy Rockett offers, "Hello cristina you should try apricot kernels do the research if your not sure but I'm convinced nothing works better," and one named Vermillion J writes, "Please research RICK SIMPSON and his HEMP OIL. Many people have testified that this oil has cured their cancers within months after they started taking the oil. Watch the film on Youtube 'Run From The Cure.'" Charlie R writes, "May I suggest something? Cancer can only live in a low pH environment. You should drink alkaline water, as it has a high pH and may help you greatly," and the user bluewaterrider writes, "Christina. Please type in UC Television Vitamin D cancer in the YouTube search box. Examine the videos. 75% reduction in mortality rate in some cases. Also, get 2nd opinions. Doctors are NOT equally knowledgeable, nor will all give you the advice you need. If you're REALLY disciplined, also look up Keto-genic Diet." A commenter named gmasters writes, "You should really research and consider dry fasting or urine therapy. These have been known to make childs play out of cancer."

I've never seen a real pink ribbon in the context of breast cancer. I've seen no silks or grosgrains, only representations of pink ribbons made of and on something else: a massive chalk drawing of a pink ribbon in a parking lot, a sticker of a pink ribbon on a car dealership window, a ribbon shape assembled from dyed martial arts belts on display in the surgeon's office, pink tinsel ribbon shapes on a silver tinsel tree, ribbons printed onto shirts and socks, ribbons airbrushed on the sides of cop cars and trash dumpsters, enameled ribbons on silver chains.

The activist Charlotte Haley, whose grandmother, sister, and daughter all had breast cancer, is credited by some for creating the first ribbon—a real one—for breast cancer in 1990. According to Breast Cancer Action, "To each packet of five ribbons she attached a postcard that read: 'The National Cancer Institute's annual budget is $1.8 billion, only 5 percent goes for cancer prevention. Help us wake up legislators and America by wearing this ribbon.'" Haley distributed these cards wherever she could, requesting no donations, spreading her campaign by word of mouth.[13]

When *Self* magazine and the Estée Lauder corporation approached Haley for a marketing partnership, the now-well-known story is that she refused to help them, saying they were too commercial. The Estée Lauder corporation did not let Haley's refusal stop them, however, and on the advice of their legal team, altered the ribbon color from peachy pink to classic pink, handing out more than a million pink ribbons in the fall of 1992. By 1993, Avon, Estée Lauder, and the Susan G. Komen breast cancer charity were all selling pink ribbon products. By 1996, breast cancer was declared, as a corporate charity recipient, "hot."[14]

On Coopdizzle's YouTube page there is an autoplay introductory video of her son laughing. Coopdizzle has written in its description: "Just Kayden being silly. I needed to clear space off my iPod lol." She follows this with a request that viewers stop suggesting treatments. "This part of my journey," she writes, "is my final journey."

Coopdizzle, who was in her thirties when she died, was diagnosed with triple-negative breast cancer the same year that I was, 2014. I began to follow her videos in the first weeks of my illness. We had similar diagnoses and similar courses of treatments: neoadjuvant chemotherapy with surgery after. My treatment worked and hers didn't, and there is no way to know how or why. Diagnosed in March 2014, by May 2015, Coopdizzle was told her cancer had returned. She died in December 2016 and spent her last months of life as a metastatic breast cancer activist, writing about her experience, talking to the media, organizing with others for collective action, and lobbying, among other things, for death with dignity and against a pink ribbon and breast cancer "awareness" culture that profits off of the continued suffering of the sick.

Coopdizzle's commitment to activism lives beyond her, including in this public post that remains pinned at the top of her Facebook page:

> First it's not about THE ribbon. It's about the Komen. It's about the fact that when the REAL Susan passed from metastatic breast cancer her sister said she would help find a cure. 30 years later we are no better off, in fact it's gotten a bit worse. SGK only donates a very small amount to the research of terminal breast cancer. They shove us under the rug and act like we aren't real. They profit off your donations and have mansions and very nice cars.

Susan G. Komen for the Cure, the world's largest breast cancer charity, began in 1982, and in 2016, according to its financial statements, raised almost $211 million for breast cancer awareness and research, and has raised $956 million to date. Komen for the Cure, which sponsors the popular Race for the Cure fund-raisers, has also conducted a robust public relations campaign against the criticism directed at it by breast cancer activists.

Komen for the Cure tells a different story about the genesis of the pink ribbon. According to the Komen version, called "The Pink Ribbon Story": "Susan G. Komen for the Cure® has used the color pink since its inception in 1982. The first Komen Race for the Cure® logo design was an abstract female runner outlined with a pink ribbon and was used during the mid 1980s through early 1990s." *Self* and Estée Lauder joined in the effort in 1992, according to Komen. Charlotte Haley's peach ribbons are not admitted into the story.[15]

The Komen foundation once partnered with KFC for "Buckets for the Cure," which sold fried chicken in large pink buckets. In 2011, the Komen foundation also marketed a perfume on the Home Shopping Network called "Promise Me," which the activist Breast Cancer Action pointed out contained the potentially carcinogenic ingredients of coumarin, oxybenzone, toluene, and galaxolide. Komen agreed to reformulate the perfume, but denied that the perfume contained harmful materials.[16] During the first Pinktober after Coopdizzle and I were diagnosed with breast cancer, 2014, Komen's CEO, Judith Salerno, earned a salary of $420,000. Also in 2014, the Baker Hughes corporation partnered with Komen to produce a thousand breast-cancer-pink fracking drills. As Karuna Jagger, president of Breast Cancer Action, said, "When future generations have to choose between safe drinking water and developing breast cancer, they can look back and thank Baker Hughes and Susan G. Komen."[17]

On Coopdizzle's Facebook page, Coopdizzle's partner describes the process of her death: "I can feel it—her burning desire to just live. I want so badly to give that to her. If only I could. If only I could."

"It's a scary place," Coopdizzle once wrote, "inside cancer land."

Nelene Fox, a schoolteacher in California, was diagnosed with breast cancer in 1991 at the age of forty. She requested that her health insurance company cover what appeared to be a promising new treatment—a bone marrow transplant with high-dose chemotherapy. They refused. Although she was able to raise private funds to cover the treatment, she died two years after her diagnosis. Her brother took the health insurance company to court, and Fox's family was awarded $89 million in damages.[18] Eighty-six other cases were filed, and forty-seven were successful. Four state legislatures mandated that the treatment be covered. Buoyed by the success of AIDS activism, women with breast cancer began an aggressive lobby for access to this new treatment. Hospitals billed the highly profitable procedure at between $80,000 and $100,000, with a cost to the hospital of less than $60,000. Health insurers began to reluctantly acquiesce, and eventually more than 41,000 breast cancer patients were given the treatment.

Researchers, doctors, and patients made optimistic claims, widely quoted in the media, that this treatment might finally be the cure. The process was long and painful, and involved isolating patients in hospital rooms for days. Side effects included sepsis, hemorrhagic cystitis, bone marrow insufficiency, pulmonary failure, veno-occlusive disease, cardiac failure, cardiac toxicity, acute myelogenous leukemia or myelodysplastic syndrome, nephrotoxicity, psychosexual disorders, and heightened vulnerability to opportunistic infections in the first year after treatment. According to some accounts, one in five women died of the treatment.[19]

The only study with conclusive data supporting this treatment for breast cancer was conducted by Dr. Werner Bezwoda in South Africa. When U.S. researchers duplicated Bezwoda's procedure on six women, four of them came away with serious heart damage. For two of them the heart damage was fatal. Another died right away of breast cancer. The fourth lived, but was disabled. The research was, Bezwoda later admitted, fraudulent.[20] More than 40,000 women endured an expensive, debilitating, life-threatening treatment that was a lie based on lies. Metastatic breast cancer still has no cure.

In 2014, the year I was diagnosed, there were an estimated 3,327,552 people with breast cancer in the United States. In 2019, the year I am finishing this book, an estimated 271,270 people will be newly diagnosed with breast cancer, and 42,260 will die of it. In the United States, breast cancer death rates slowly increased every year until 1975, held steady until 1989, and then began to decrease after that, except in the case of patients younger than fifty, whose death rates have been relatively level since 2007.

Who dies from the collection of diseases called "breast cancer" is influenced by income, education, gender, family status, access to health care, race, and age. Black women have both a lower rate of being diagnosed with breast cancer and a higher rate of mortality from it. Unmarried women have a greater risk of dying from their breast cancer, too, and of not receiving adequate care for it. Breast cancer patients who live in poor neighborhoods have a lower survival rate at every stage of diagnosis. Unmarried breast cancer patients who live in poor neighborhoods have the lowest survival rate of all. Some people with breast cancer, like those who are transgender or people who are single parents, at the writing of this book haven't yet made it into their own epidemiological category.

These are statistics, but they are not always truths. It is, in fact, difficult to get any sense of the scope of breast cancer or the accuracy of the available numbers. This is not only because there are sometimes profit and public relations motives behind epidemiological accounts of breast cancer—for example, breast cancer charities sometimes present the numbers as telling an optimistic story of medical progress—but because surveillance technologies have increasingly uncovered physiological occurrences that have been understood to be breast cancer when they weren't. There is no way of knowing how many people have been led to believe they had breast cancer when they instead had benign conditions that were no threat to their lives. The good news is that researchers and oncology practitioners have begun in the past few years to seriously address the problem of breast cancer overdiagnosis and overtreatment and the disabling effect it has on people's lives.

People diagnosed with DCIS—a condition some call "Stage 0" breast cancer, with which an estimated 63,960 people were diagnosed in 2018—frequently report that their doctors told them that their breasts were "ticking time bombs." Some with DCIS have opted for mastectomy or other forms of aggressive, expensive treatment. The problem is that people with DCIS appear to have no greater chance of breast cancer than those without it. People's bodies are made of cells, not time bombs, but there is no billion-dollar industry devoted to reminding us of that.

In October 2016, a study published in the *New England Journal of Medicine* confirmed earlier research about breast cancer overtreatment and led the *Los Angeles Times* to declare that the majority of women diagnosed with breast cancer via mammography received unnecessary treatment. Early detection did not, as the saying went, save lives, but instead, damaged them, costing billions of dollars and resulting in life-altering effects. As the UCLA breast cancer specialist Dr. Patricia Ganz is quoted as saying, "If we just keep doing what we've been doing, we're exposing lots of people to treatment they don't need or can't afford."[21]

Millions of people have breast cancer, except when they don't; many others think they are survivors of the disease despite research now designating them victims of medical surveillance, instead; lack of access to treatment harms, access to treatment harms; surveillance harms, lack of surveillance harms; researchers fake cures, patients fake cancer, and doctors do, too. "What If," a *Mother Jones* headline asks about the crisis, "Everything Your Doctors Told You About Breast Cancer Was Wrong?"[22]

The novelist Kathy Acker's breast cancer most likely couldn't have been cured by chemotherapy, but she had no way of knowing this when she refused chemotherapy in 1996. Or at least she had no rational way to know this. She did, however, appear to have another way to know it. "I live as I believe," wrote Acker in "The Gift of Disease," "that belief is equal to the body."[23]

Some of her friends, however—despite lack of evidence— seem certain that her decision to forgo chemotherapy was the cause of her death. That Acker "wanted" to die or somehow brought about her own death is one of the many durable untruths in circulation about breast cancer. Sarah Schulman, in her book *The Gentrification of the Mind*, writes that Acker died of "bad treatment decisions regarding her breast cancer."[24] In an account of Acker's death published in *Hazlitt* magazine, Ira Silverberg claimed it was "certain she wanted to die" and that "it was her exit strategy."[25]

Acker did not merely, as was written in the *Financial Times*, "refuse chemotherapy because her alternative healers assured her the cancer was gone."[26] She refused chemotherapy for a complex set of reasons, including fear of chemotherapy, cost of treatment, and her doctor's statement that chemotherapy would only raise her chance of recurrence 20 percent. Had Acker agreed to one of the regimens of chemotherapy available in 1996, it would have almost certainly meant the last months of her life would have been spent with some variation of the following: dry itchy eyes, skin lesions, anal lesions, mouth lesions, a bloody nose, wasted muscles, dying nerves, rotting teeth, no hair or immune system, too brain-damaged to write, throwing up, losing her memory, losing her vocabulary, and severely fatigued. These are the most common side effects, but there are others, too, including blood clots, heart failure, and chemo-therapy-induced leukemia—and still more, like a risk of deadly pneumonia and hospital-borne infections. Acker would have most likely endured some or all of this while also enduring the cascading physical symptoms of her cancer itself.

Given that her cancer metastasized quickly to her liver and lungs, and that her doctor did not offer her the option of tamoxifen, which was available at the time, it is probably safe to conclude that Acker's cancer was hormone-receptor-negative, either what we now call triple negative, or what had a more severe prognosis at the time, hormone-receptor-negative breast cancer with Her2 sensitivity. Using the survival rates provided to her by her physician along with her own description of her diagnosis, I entered her disease's statistics into LifeMath, the prognosis database, which I used to make decisions about the treatment of my own. A cancer like Acker's, one that killed her in eighteen months, had a similar two-year death rate whether or not a patient underwent chemotherapy. According to the results, five people out of one hundred with this type of cancer will die within two years with chemotherapy; around the same number would die without. Some studies have suggested that an initial round of chemotherapy can speed up aggressive cancers like hers, introducing the possibility that any treatment might have even hastened death. There wasn't a cure then. There isn't one now. In making a principled judgment to live according to her values, Acker did the best anyone could do.

Maybe medical historians will view chemotherapy with the same perplexed curiosity that ours do formerly common medical practices such as bloodletting—that not only did we severely poison people in attempts to make them well, but that even in those instances when chemotherapy doesn't and won't work and results in death, damage, and disability, there remains a popular desire for breast cancer patients to undergo it. When it isn't motivated by profit, this overtreatment seems to result from superstition rather than science, and the irrational desire for chemotherapy isn't just aroused in the loved ones of a cancer patient, as it was in Acker's case. It sometimes occurs in cancer patients themselves. There are patients who, out of fear, convention, misinformation, or social pressure, undergo chemotherapy even in circumstances where it has no particular medical use and no science to support it. It is as if the world itself is captivated by the unholy rites of the infusion room and the sentimental dramas of lost hair, wasting limbs, weakened women. Chemotherapy's cultural spell is so strong that people without cancer sometimes see patients deciding to forgo it as an excuse to abandon the sick. "I lost a lot of friends," Acker said, who "couldn't bear to watch."[27]

Instead of opting for the painful death that she was offered by the available medicine, what Kathy Acker did was what she said she wanted to do with the remainder of her life after diagnosis: Live. Refusal can be isolating; the social enforcement of medical compliance around a gendered disease like breast cancer, brutal. As Acker wrote: "Many of my friends phoned me, crying and yelling at me for not undergoing chemotherapy."[28] But despite how everything in the world seems set up to kill a woman before she is actually dead, Kathy Acker chose not to. She waited to die until her end was irrefutable, and even then, according to accounts of her friends, tried, at least for good measure, to refute it.[29] Breast cancer killed Kathy Acker. Kathy Acker did not kill Kathy Acker.

Cancer kills people, as does treatment, as does lack of treatment, and what anyone believes or feels has nothing to do with it. I could hold every right idea, exhibit every virtue, do every good deed, and follow every institutional command and still die of breast cancer, or I could believe and do every wrong thing and still live.

Dying of breast cancer is not evidence of the weakness or moral failure of the dead. The moral failure of breast cancer is not in the people who die: it is in the world that makes them sick, bankrupts them for a cure that also makes them sick, then, when the cure fails, blames them for their own deaths.

As Coopdizzle, who was thirty-four when she died, has tagged in the corner of her posthumous YouTube video a warning: "Please do not say I lost my battle."

As Audre Lorde, who also refused chemotherapy for breast cancer, wrote ten years before Acker's diagnosis:

I warn myself, don't even pretend not to say no, loudly and often, no matter how symbolically. Because the choices presented in our lives are never simple or fable-clear. Survival never presents itself as "do this particular thing precisely as directed and you will go on living. Don't do that and no question about it you will surely die." Despite what the doctor said, it just doesn't happen that way.[30]

4.

Now that I am undying, the world is full of possibility. I could write a book in which nothing is left out, or write a work of undying literature in which everything that is missing shows up as the shadow of its own shape, or one where nothing could be displayed except as its consequence. Nothing would be missing from this book where nothing is not permitted: not the material world nor all of its semi-material relations. We do not often know the source of the things of the world and so are mostly left to imagine their lineage. We are abandoned by cause, left to guess at the effect, and in our guesses, we are abandoned by truth, left only to error, permitted metaphysics but never really wanting them in the first place.

Karl Marx wrote, "All that is solid melts into air," which is true, as it is also true that all that is air becomes, under a later version of those same conditions, too polluted to breathe. We imagine that this air could fall on us as rain, and that as it is also in us, it falls away from us as tears and sweat and urine. Respiration is a refeeding of what is abstract into what is so tangible it changes our form, at least slightly. Then it dissipates, again, we never know as what. As one of the undying I will now try to conjure up not the undying soul but instead an undying substance, reground the atmospheric as new evidence.

The same technologies of thought that humans once used to understand our souls are now what it takes to understand a Baby Shrek figurine from the dollar store. The human world has never required an instrument so vast.

IN THE TEMPLE OF GIULIETTA MASINA'S TEARS

Also, while the said creature was occupied with
the writing of this treatise, she had many holy
tears and much weeping, and often there came
a flame of fire about her breast, very hot and
delectable . . .

—*The Book of Margery Kempe*, 1501

1.

Before I got sick, I'd been making plans for a place for public weeping, hoping to install in major cities an almost-religious monument where anyone who needed it could get together to cry in good company and with the proper equipment. It would be like God's Tabernacle in Exodus, a precisely imagined architecture of shared sadness: gargoyles made of night sweat, moldings made of longest minutes, support beams made of *I-can't-go-on-I-must-go-on*. I would call this *The Temple of Giulietta Masina's Tears* after the Italian actress who plays Cabiria, an aging sex worker in the Fellini film who cries while swept into a parade of young people after her false-true love, Giorgio, tries to push her off a cliff and steal her money. The walls of the temple would have a projection of Masina as Cabiria weeping while almost smiling; there'd be a looped soundtrack of Judy Garland's voice breaking on that mournful outtake of "Over the Rainbow." When planning the temple, I remembered the existence of the people who have hated those they call *crybabies*, how they might respond with rage to a public place in which crying strangers gathered en masse to cry about whatever they liked. Foreclosing this potential danger was part

of the formal problem: how to make a space for the physical expression of both singular and common sorrow, a
place that both comfortably exposed suffering as what
is shared and that guaranteed some protection against
anti-sadness reactionaries. It would have been something tremendous to trick those who would freely inflict extra pain on people already in pain into their own
private-hell chambers, and at the same time to offer pain's
sufferers the exquisite comforts of stately public marble
troughs in which to collectivize their tears. But I never did
this. Later, when I was sick, I was on a chemotherapy drug
with a side effect of endless crying, tears dripping without agency from my eyes no matter what I was feeling
or where I was. I called this *the season of Cartesian
weeping*—the months my body's sadness disregarded
my mind's attempts to convince me I was okay—and I
cried every minute, whether I was sad or not, my self a
mobile, embarrassed public monument of tears. I didn't
need to build the temple for weeping, then, having been
one. I've just always hated it when anyone suffers alone.

2.

As if pain were the opposite of beauty, I walked through the decorative-arts wings of a museum taking notes on how to turn the cancer pavilion's IV poles into beaux arts chandeliers, how chemo bags could look like kaleidoscopic Grecian urns, how the endless feelings-less weeping of a chemotherapy patient could be done in the service of ornate lacrimal vessels and poisonous irrigation schemes.

This is a treatise on pain made of notes and starts: ephemeral sensation's monument of an ephemeralist's half-literature. I've been keeping a list of subtitles for it, such as: *mutilated body as ecopoetic, unbearable pain as Kantian critique, dolor plastico, eros-absentia, pain's paradoxical democracy, a formal feeling sums, every pietà a mastectomy scar, bionegated social unremittingest, etiological epithetics, oncosurrealism, suture as epic theory, the somapathetic fallacy of spring—*

> from *Zoonomia, or the Laws of Organic Life, 1794*:
> "compassion is the pain we experience at the sight of misery"

from my journals: "unwaning woe"

from Twitter: "can you imagine an essay with the
    motion of ruins?"

from Alphonse Daudet's *In the Land of Pain*, 1888:
    "Pain, you must be everything for me. Let me find
    in you all those foreign lands you will not let me
    visit. Be my philosophy, be my science."

I wanted to write about pain without any philosophy. I wanted to describe an education in pain and that education's political uses. But in literature, pain mostly excludes literature. And in the available politics, pain is often just what moves us to plead for its end.

True/False:
1. In philosophy, pain is a feather plucked from its bird.
2. In literature, pain is an index separated from its book.
3. In movies, pain is a tree, but never its ax.

There's a rumor that any consideration of pain nests under phenomenology, but phenomenology mostly stops at a modest sliver of available pain and declares it a universal whole. "My body" gets turned into "the body" there. Emotional pain overruns the physical, as if it isn't actually the other way around, as if it isn't pain in our bodies or its absence determining what kind of day or hour or minute we have, whether or how we work, whether or how we breathe or sleep or love. Then the already apparently abstract goes floating away into further abstraction, like a dust particle submitted to a discourse made of dust.

To be a minor person in great pain at this point in history is to be a person who feels inside their body when most people just want to look.

There's expository pain like an X-ray machine, illuminating the difficult mysteries of the interior. There's the pain that becomes metaphor and there's the pain that's read as if it's the canon. Then there's trash pain—the libertine pain of malingering, which is more like a texture than an image. Then there's the epic pain of a cure.

If this were a work of philosophy, I would argue that the spectacle of pain is what keeps us from understanding it, that what we see of pain is inadequate to what we can know, that a problem with understanding pain at this point in history is the generalizing effect and market saturation of vision, but I am 1) not a philosopher and 2) don't really know.

My pain's naked grammar was:

how doe sone go on like htis the days gone finally in a way that can't be though I have a light on my face to hceer me and I took an advicl will take more take vitamin d fake every sunlight the world on fire last night while I slept in such rgitheous pain

True/False:

1. As pain incapacitates a person, it also incapacitates the dictionary.
2. Pain is an ugly gathering of adjectives.
3. Any word for pain is always in a language we cannot yet understand.

A widely held notion about pain seems to be that it "destroys language."[1] But pain doesn't destroy language: it changes it. What is difficult is not impossible. That English lacks an adequate lexicon for all that hurts doesn't mean it always will, just that the poets and marketplaces that have invented our dictionaries have not—when it comes to suffering—done the necessary work.

Suppose for a moment the claims about pain's ineffability are historically specific and ideological, that pain is widely declared inarticulate for the reason that we are not supposed to share a language for how we really feel.

An example of this assertion about the ineffability of pain is found in Hannah Arendt's *The Human Condition*, in which she describes pain as "the most private and least communicable" of all experience. She goes on to write that pain is "the true borderline experience between life as 'being among men' . . . and death," claiming that its subjectivity is so intense that pain has no appearance. Contrast this philosophical truism about pain's lack of communicability with your own experience of witnessing another living creature in pain. The howls, cries, screams, shrieks, and whimpers of another in pain are unequivocal. The words "that hurts!" or "I am in pain" or "that burns" or "this aches," and various exclamations like "ow!" and "ouch!" and "motherfucker!" are also generally undeniable communications of pain. A dog or cat in pain is equally communicative. The look of a face in pain—even a non-human face—cannot be mistaken for a look of contentment. Winces, agonized expressions, leaking tears, and gnashed teeth are so communicative, for example, that "a pained expression" is a common turn of phrase.

The drive to stop the pain of others because pain is so loud, so vividly expressed, often takes the form of wanting to do anything at all to end the pain of another precisely because of the way that this pain inflicts the experience of an impossible-to-bear sympathetic discomfort—sometimes in the form of annoyance, sometimes in the form of anxiety, sometimes in the form of pity—upon one's self. This drive to end the immediate pain of another creature in one's own proximity is so strong that it can sometimes compel the witness to pain to inflict greater pain upon the sufferer, as when adults threaten to give children "something to cry about" in order to make them quiet. Pain is so communicative, in fact, that the source of much violence could well be found in reaction to pain's hyperexpressivity. It is the clearness of pain that gives sadists their reward. If pain were silent and hidden, there would be no incentive for its infliction. Pain, indeed, is a condition that creates *excessive* appearance. Pain is a fluorescent feeling.

That pain is incommunicable is a lie in the face of the near-constant, trans-species, and universal communicability of pain. So the question, finally, is not whether pain has a voice or appearance: the question is whether those people who insist that it does not are interested in what pain has to say, and whose bodies are doing the talking. Jean-Jacques Rousseau, who believed that "commiseration must be so much the more energetic, the more intimately the animal" part of human nature, theorized that a lack of response to those in pain is a characteristic unique to philosophers. "It is philosophy," he writes in *A Discourse Upon the Origin and the Foundation of Equality*, "that destroys [a person's] communications with other men; it is in consequence of her dictates that he mutters to himself at the sight of another in distress, 'You may perish for aught I care, nothing can hurt me.' Nothing less than those evils, which threaten the whole species, can disturb the calm sleep of the philosopher."

On the Internet, pain is a series of bulletin board posts about hermeneutics and time.

Julian Teppe began his pain-positive Dolorist movement with his 1935 *Apologie pour l'anormal*, or "Dolorist Manifesto." Teppe argues against the tyranny of the healthy, and makes an argument for pain as an education, liberating a person from materiality and providing an opportunity for clarity. "I consider extreme anguish," wrote Teppe, "particularly that of somatic origin, as the perfect incitement for developing pure idealism."[2]

Sometimes to make a hero of one's pain is pain's only course, but even so, pain's education should be in more than in pain's valorization.

I imagined a body-tourism or soma-exchange support system in which a person could temporarily inhabit the sensorium of a person in pain. On a scale of 1 to 10 you could feel

1. the delicate raw and anxious pain of fingernails and toenails lifting away from their beds
2. the dense agonizing pain of bones expanding as they fill up with artificially stimulated blood cells
3. the pillowy congested pain of the inflamed body in contact with the mattress
4. the heavy exhausted pain of the clothes that hang on the pathologically sensate body
5. the inside-out surprise pain of needles puncturing arms, chest, fatty thigh, outside hand, inside wrist, also of IVs
6. the searing spreading pain of painful drugs dispersing
7. the alien to-do-list pain of subdermally implanted devices against the muscle and skin
8. or the zapping electrical apocalypse of dying-nerve-ending pain

9. or the raw openness of mouth-sores pain; the patient, etiologically blank-faced hurting pain of poison-swollen ligaments, teeth, tendons, joints, and muscles; the corrosive pain of drug-induced cellular suicide; the expansive aching itching pain of dying hair follicles, etc. etc. etc.
10. the panicking inadequacies of all genres, a new crisis of transmission—

To invite you to my body in pain might have been more like an invitation to a seminar in dimensional shift. In pain, the spatial becomes temporal, as in *pain is the experience of a location that exists only as desperation for its end.*

It was easy to get caught up in seeing the world as a scheme to discipline the senses and the feelings and thoughts brought around by them, to think the world is a boiling pot, kept down only by a great lie's lid, to hope, too, that the answer is to learn to feel differently, sense otherwise, think in a new way, and the lid will pop off, the water of truth overrun its container of ideology: *oh there*, I guess, like we could critique ourselves free.

But I believed in the dirt, having never put my hands in the ether: blood up, not stars down, also *limbic materialism, lacrimonial feminism, violence as the negative education of the senses, herds, the arrangement of the earth its materials and substances environments and objects, what is ours and how to get it, transmutation—seepage, anti-enlightenment enlightenmentarians, under-histories, reading wrong, everything that is but that is barely perceptible as such, black dresses on broomsticks, violability, literature as it allows for maximum epistemological possibility . . .*

We can't think ourselves free, but that's no reason not to get an education.

I wanted to make a clinic fable, and then to make it monumental, as if a lesson in having a body could be installed on a government lawn.

First there's the needle everyone knows hurts, but everyone in charge says doesn't. Then there's the needle everyone knows can't hurt, but someone who has been through some stuff still feels.

the first needle:

People in chemotherapy are often prescribed anesthetic cream to apply over their chemotherapy ports. The numbing cream is intended to make the insertion of the large needle into a patient's chest bearable. Perhaps the numbing cream insures that the insertion hurts less, but the insertion still hurts. "It hurts," I'd tell the nurses when they would always tell me otherwise, they who have put their faith in a cream. "It really does," I'd say. "You put a large needle into my chest," I'd remind them as they would tell me the needle was painless (or "a pressure") while my body reacted visibly with pain. The chemotherapy room in which I began treatment was open: all the sick and all who attended to them could stare at each other with the sick becoming sicker and therefore, in the perverse logic of cancer treatment, better. "You're right," said a fellow patient, a woman, watching. "It really does hurt," said a man surrounded by his adult children, all of us in the infusion room then all joining together to say what appears to hurt actually *does hurt* so that no one would ever again say while they were hurting us that what really hurt us—hurt all of us—never did.

the second needle:

I tried to believe in science, but I could still feel the pain. I closed my eyes, asked the nurse not to tell me *when*, but each time the skin over my chest was punctured by the needle, my body startled and I yelped. Tissue-expander breast reconstruction is widely regarded as very painful, the kind of process that requires you to sign consent forms for your future opiate addiction. But the known pain of breast reconstruction is a long, tedious pain, felt less at the clinic than outside of it a day or two after each expansion procedure intended to stretch muscle and skin. The particular pain I was feeling, the one of the needle going into the subdermal metal ports of the hard plastic expanders that had been surgically implanted after my double mastectomy under my splayed-open pectoral muscles, was an immediate kind that was supposed to be impossible. The nerves in my chest had been cut during the mastectomy: the ones near my skin should have been dead, were dead, the doctors told me, in 99 percent of everyone else. The doctors and other workers in the office believed my pain because they could see it, having me close my eyes to test it, trying to trick me about the puncture of each needle. No one could explain it, having never seen an impossible and unscientific pain like it before. Medical students came in to watch my expanders being filled, watched an impossible pain (my impossible pain) in action, to see my pain for themselves. The pain I felt in my chest each weekly session was a clever ghost, I guess, a phantom sensation with a memory so thorough that it could react to unfelt infliction with total precision in matters of space and time.

Every amputation is subject to the same ghostly way of living ever after, the potential feeling of the nevermore of the phantom "I miss." My lost body parts were invisible sites of sympathy with the visible world. Acts of violence, representations of acts of violence, a wince, or a hurt look on someone else's face created the mirror sensation in the parts of me that no longer existed. In what wasn't anymore, I felt anyone else's. A comic pratfall could do it, filmic shoot-outs, a student with disgruntled feelings, a person complaining on Twitter, an exhausted worker, someone stubbing her toes, news of ISIS, news of drones, news of the police.[3]

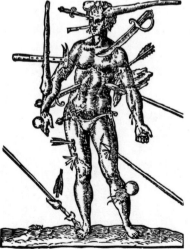

My version of being a thinker then was *although my right arm hurt and I didn't know why, my chest hurt and I did.* My pain had its reasons when I was sick; that is, pain was my body being *reasonable.* I'd been cut into, poisoned, harvested, amputated, implanted, punctured, weakened, and severely infected, often all at once. And for this reason of the *reasonableness* of my pain, I knew I should distinguish my life in pain from the pain life of the tortured. But torture has its reasons, too, like the existence of the metaphor "the body politic" and the perniciousness of that figure when it has extracting information as its cure. Torturers always claim that torture itself is reasonable, torturing out security or freedom or god or righteousness or other suspicious rhetorics, but I can't imagine that when torturers mean something by inflicting pain it reduces the feeling in the tortured of being maximally hurt. A cancer patient can tell herself why what is done to her must be done, but this does not often fix the feeling that she has been cut up, poisoned, harvested, amputated, implanted, punctured, weakened, and infected, often all at once. And as torture is pain instrumentalized by an extra-distortion of time—part of torture's effectiveness is the lie that it might never end—cancer treatment is so often pain de-instrumentalized inside the extra-distortion of time that is called "dying." Cancer treatment sometimes ends well, of course, as mine did, so sometimes it only feels unending, but it also has a stubborn chronicity, since for so many people it can go on forever, which means at least until they are dead.

Every time I was asked to give pain a number, my friends and I made plans to sneak pamphlets with alternate vocabularies of pain into the waiting rooms. These guides to the new language of pain would consist mostly of the poems of Emily Dickinson. How does your pain feel on a scale of 1 to 10?

```
341 After Great Pain—A Formal Feeling
    comes x
477 No man can compass despair x
584 It ceased to hurt me x
599 There is a pain so utter x
650 Pain has an Element of Blank x
761 From Blank to Blank x
1049 Pain has but one acquaintance and
    that is death
```

In this dream, I was at a therapist's office for people who had parts of corpses in them. The therapy was not for the person with the corpse inside her, but for the corpse itself. The corpse in me had been through a lot: her chest had been used as a radiator, parts of her had traveled on the back of a truck, she had been in some seedy places, she was played with like a toy. I only had a few square inches of her in me, but the pain and swelling in my body made it clear what I was rejecting. Life-Cell (corporate vision: "surgery without complications") brands the sterilized cadaver skin[4] used as a sling for breast implants as "Alloderm," but hygienic nominalism could do nothing to afford how this fraction of a dead person implanted in me filled the dream life of April 2015 with a wide and recurring version of a cadaver's terror.

Sometimes I would call myself a "sick person," and I would think of everyone else, if they weren't sick, as "future sick persons." I would also sometimes think of the arrangement of the world as those who were currently sick and those who thought they were well, but to place each person in these categories wasn't so easy. I had been, I am sure, sick before I knew it. If disease is a space, and if pain is a duration, neither could be an identity.

Chemotherapy is death-against-death modernism. Surgery is the Enlightenment. Reconstruction is the phase that escapes periodization—medicine against absence—not growing crops but the appearance of crops on recently salted fields. Disability is whatever isn't history, a battleground turned into a 7-Eleven on which someone has graffitied PAIN WITHOUT VICTORY.[5]

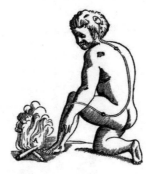

The philosopher Emmanuel Levinas wrote that the least one could say about suffering was that it is "for nothing." That it is "for nothing" is also what people say about poetry.

If suffering is like a poem, I want mine to be lurid, righteous, and goth.

When asked to draw pain, my students make mostly inchoate scribbles, derivative diagrams learned from aspirin ads, or punctuation marks.

An exclamation point is useful, but pain can also be described by its duration, its magnitude, its locations, its relations, its variations, its disruptions, its histories, its temperatures, its haptics, its memories, its patterns, its pressures, its sympathies, its forms, its purposes, its references, its causes, its economics, its forgettings, its dimensions, its categories, its effects.

Amnesia is vice-president to pain and the mother of philosophy. What philosophy often forgets is this: that few of us exist most of the time as just one person. This un-oneness can hurt, just like any oneness can hurt, too.

We move in and out of each other's holes or make new ones. We cut each other open, leave wasted bits of DNA around, leave shards of evolutionary codices discarded in our lovers and our mothers and our children. Many of us have bodies that other people have sometimes lived or died in, too. It can hurt that we enter and exit, are entered and left, that we are born into another sentient other's hands and into the environment more sentient others built around us, born into the rest in the world, all capable of pain, too, which will make us hurt even more.

A reminder of our un-oneness is at least one counterpurpose of literature. This is why I tried to write down pain's leaky democracies, the shared vistas of the terribly felt.

Before my education in it, pain had been local, the simple pain of a simple life, that humble pain of the partial, the kind of ordinary pain of the minor that would lead a person to believe that there are such things as organs or limbs or identities.

My new calamity meant it was possible to feel every cell at once and, in these, every mitochondrion, and that it was possible, too, to have a millionfold shitshow of sensations in locations newly realized, and that also these sensations were conspiring toward the knowledge that something called something like an "arm" is a lie to obscure its actuality as a city or a war or an avalanche and something called an "armpit" is a misprision of all that crumbles or a coral reef drying and something called "a body" does not end at the end of its flesh and that this disproves Europe and the Enlightenment and that something called a "metaphor" was too narrow a technique to describe the diversity and number of agonies that could now be acutely and all at once perceived.

I wanted to learn to draw maps so I could chart this. I'd publish a distinguished atlas of the infernal geographies of the interior of the body in multiple forms of pain and the cities, wars, agricultural innovations, and topological eruptions happening there.

But it would be wrong to present pain as if it were a property—as wrong as presenting pain as a metaphysics. In pain, there is always something to explore, but never anything to conquer. There's no empire in a nerve.

My education in pain was a radical materialization of sensation that some mistake for magic, to feel other people's suffering in the space of what is no longer there. That we are always alone in pain is a lie, I think: that language fails it, another. It is history that fails pain, as it also fails language, but the truth of history is also the truth of language and this is that everything will always change and soon. Every sensate body is a reminder that tomorrow is not today. Maybe suffering pain is not for nothing, or is for nothing-plus: pain's education is an education in *everything* and a reminder of *nothing's all.*

_ WASTED LIFE

-
-
-
-
—
-
-
-
—
-
-
-
—
-
-
-
—
-
-
-

I wanted to write about exhaustion the way I used to write about love. Like love, exhaustion both requires language and baffles it, and like love, it is not as if exhaustion will kill you, no matter how many times you might declare that you are dying of it.

Exhaustion is not like death, either, which has a plot and a readership. Exhaustion is boring, requires no genius, is democratic in practice, lacks fans. In this, it's like experimental literature.

I was once not exhausted, and then I was. I got sick, and then the late effects of treatment made me exhausted. I was taken to the moment of depletion and then taken past that, and after my recovery kept there in the probably forever of never-all-better, sinking further and further into exhaustion's ground. What happens if you can no longer self-repair? To be depleted is not to die: it is to barely do something else.

Exhaustion is a culmination of history presented in one body, then another, then another. If exhaustion as a subject has become newly popular it is because a once-proletarian feeling has now become a feeling of the proletarianized all.

The exhausted are always trying, even when they don't want to, even when they are too exhausted to name *trying* as *trying* or to think about it like that. The *trying* of the exhausted is fuel for the machine that keeps running them over in the first place. Life doesn't have to be happy to be long.

Trying is the method of traveling with a body through efforts to find the limit of those efforts' ends. You *just can't*, but have to. Now you will. First a breath, next an achievement, then another combination of attempts, a failure or a nap or a bad decision, all in an attempt at *attempting*, eating a high-protein afternoon snack and playing out with one's existence existing's limit-end.

The exhausted are plastic and adaptable. They bend better and more to what is necessary for their having been worn down. They live as fluidly as the water into which a corpse tied with rocks has been plunged or into which a ship sank or from which a dolphin surfaced.

The exhausted have a desire: to no longer be exhausted. The exhausted can have this one desire, to no longer be exhausted, as the prerequisite for the possibility of again having many desires, to no longer be exhausted so that they can want something other, to want what they really want, which is to no longer be exhausted, so that their bodies can offer the possibility again of love or art or pleasure, of thinking without regretting, of achievement, too, or something beyond failed and sorrowful trying at the *barely*.

Our wanting is not our wanting, exactly, when it is exposed like this through being too tired to want anything. What the exhausted once believed was a desire from inside them showed itself to be a desire from what was outside, what had been there before them and what was ordered by whatever wasn't them.

But it's not that abstract, energy and lack of it; and not that abstract, being too worn out to want anything but to not be worn out anymore; and not that abstract, the hyperfocused forever of not having enough of any life to do with it what one could. The exhausted are exhausted because they sell the hours of their lives to survive their lives, then they use the hours they haven't sold to get their lives ready for selling, and the hours after that to do the same for the other lives they love.

A person can be anything, she is told, *if she puts her mind to it* in the economic zone of unfettered personal possibility. It's the free trade of souls across the open borders of indefatigability. It's a series of horizon-wide choices unlimited by limitations except for how all possibilities will be circumscribed by the capacity to exhaust oneself to discover a possibility's end.

Fate was shipwrecked, so in its place, they sent us agency. Free to love, free to work, free to get, free to enter multiple and contractual and subcontractual realms in which each element of a person's existence is negotiated to the effect of determining her position only by how it wears her out.

In this version of freedom, the invisibility of all fences is the point of every invisible fence. The apparent lack of limits among the limits mystifies both limits and limitlessness. There are horizons that sink, roads and highways that seem to go on for as long as one has the capacity to travel them, and then, at the place at which it wears you out, you find a real fence.

Freedom ends exactly there, hung up on your own system's failure, a former dynamo that is now an evaporated animal, all free energy having been expended freely in a quest toward freedom's end.

The exhausted rise each day, or at least most of them do. That they rise most days is testament to the distance between how a person feels and what they do.

A person can and often does rise in a *will-optional* attempt at getting out of bed, and when they can't rise, it's almost never from lack of wanting to. No matter how much they *just can't*, the exhausted, if they are living, continue to. They continue to, like everyone who does until they don't anymore, but they continue to more miserably than those who are not exhausted yet. To live and so to eat, drink water, to find a method—work or love—by which to afford to eat, to pay their bills and pay their taxes, to use the bathroom, to put on clothes, to care for their loved ones, requires that they rise, at least sometimes. The exhausted might almost do what they are supposed to do, but as a consequence of their depletion, they almost never do what they want. The exhausted don't die. Or if they do die, it is only once, like everyone else, and from anything. An exhausted body almost always provides the wrong information. The wrong information is also the right information: things can't go on like this, and so they do, and what gets proved is the blurred edge between being alive and being dead.

Living takes the shape of the effort to exist. In the long night of this *effort to exist's* case file, each hour recedes into a lack of energy to achieve a measure of that hour's length. Everything is tried—that's how it gets exhausted— and a person trying to take notes on this writes, "I'm exhausted," because they are too tired to put down their pen.

That you will run out of yourself trying to make yourself is the yogic prelude to the entrepreneurial rules of existing. It's the epoch of *yes*; the age of unlimited *can*, a mass existence in the soma-pathetic fallacy of the body and earth together registering the alarming texture of our mutual expiration.

Here's an asana of auto-exploitation:

> First, a breath. Then sweating. Now sweating with breathing. Then achievement. Then email and sweating. Now breathing and achieving and emailing. Now working while breathing. Now failure and sleeping and breathing. Now refusing to sleep while breathing or attempting to refuse to breathe while still sweating and failing and achieving.

Exhaustion as a method of existing combines all actions until it finds the edges of the shape of existing's end. Like everything aleatory, as a method it has one outcome: possibility. This possibility is mostly the possibility that all things will end in exhaustion.

The exhausted find their energy wasted again. Sleep, which is often the remedy for tiredness, disappoints the exhausted. Sleep is full of the work of dreams, full of the way that sleep begets more sleep, full of the way that more sleep can beget more exhaustion, and that more exhaustion begets more exhaustion for which the remedy is almost never just sleep.

The exhausted are the saints of the wasted life, if a saint is a person who is better than others at suffering. What the exhausted suffer better is the way bodies and time are so often at odds with each other in our time of overwhelming and confused chronicity, when each hour is amplified past circadianism, quadrupled in the quarter-hour's agenda, Pomodoro-ed, hacked, FOMO-ed, and productivized. The exhausted are the human evidence of each minute misunderstood to be an empire for finance, of each human body misunderstood to be an instrument that should play a thousand compliant songs at once.

We can't measure spirit. This because it isn't real, or at least because it is not material, but it feels real when we become acutely aware of our own aridity. But no matter how potentially unalive or indistinct an exhausted person feels inside of herself, her body will look like a body, discreet, alive and animate, and capable of trying more, of trying harder, of improving or remedying or aspiring or producing.

We are never our spirits' containers. No person's body is marked with a measuring line. No one knows how boundless we once were or could be, and by looking, no one knows what it used to feel like to exist, and how different it feels to exist now, or how we were once full and are now depleted. The water is gone because the empty glass tells us so. In order to appear used up, a body has to look like a particular life's packaging, providing rough measure of its interior's resources, then its lack of them.

The exhausted person is "used up," but can't ever be seen as that, only as what is potentially (like everyone else and probably everything else in the instrumentalized world) used. The "used up" mostly belongs to substances or objects that can be or commonly are contained, and it is mostly in relationship to their container that what can be used up becomes legible as use-up-able. Probably a thing that can be "used up" can't be considered actually used until it is gone entirely, and maybe this is because a thing that can be "used up" is often a thing with a use that is recognizably metabolic, like food or soap or gasoline. The interior of the compost barrel stays dark.

The exhausted look exhausted because they aren't trying, even if what they are exhausted from is all that trying. "You look exhausted," we might say to the exhausted only when we remember them as once vital, noticing the alteration only through comparison, meaning you once looked okay but now *you look gaunt, you have circles under your eyes, your face is puffy or your features deformed, you drag and do not spring, you seem to hold your head above your shoulders with the greatest effort, what you say is not too lucid, you fly off the handle in rage, you cry too easily, your words come out jumbled, you cry and say "I'm tired" and say "I'm exhausted" and you cry because you are so tired.*

An exhausted person, trying to look less so, will *try*, as trying is what she is good at. She will put concealer under her eyes, add blush to her cheeks, do all the tricks the magazines and websites tell her will make her look less exhausted: curl her eyelashes up so that her eyelids might droop less, drink coffee, take Adderall, exercise, realize it is Tuesday, then that it is Friday, then that it is the end of the month, then that it is the beginning, then that time has rushed forward without her, carrying with it her to-do list but leaving her behind.

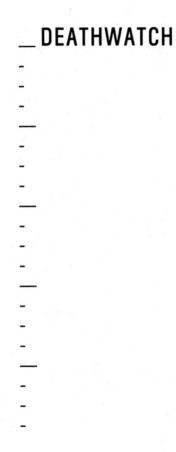

__ DEATHWATCH

It's all made up. I mean having a body in the world is not to have a body in truth: it's to have a body in history.

All is heuristic! would be my version of Ecclesiastes. We bring a tool to bear on every tool to bear. Nothing is certain but what is between us and what we need to know about: fabrication, appearance, Instagram filters, muddy forms. We make shapes in our mind to understand the world, and even then, we never quite do.

On February 14 of the year A.D. 170, Aristides dreamed he was in his hometown of Smyrna, "distrusting everything plain and visible."[1] I write in my journal: *I hope to never write beautifully if what I am saying is untrue.*

There is the condition of being the bearer of desirable suffering. Devout Christians in medieval Europe would sometimes kiss lepers. They'd put their nose in a leper's wounds or have one sleep in their bed to leave behind what they called "perfume."[2]

There is the condition of sitting very still, of moving less or hardly or not at all, and then also of the world continuing in its own motion, to be asynchronous with the world so that a day blurs into the next, then months, then years, then the motion of the world gone out of hand, never to be caught up with again.

There is the condition of feeling like a city that is most interesting for its ruins.

In *Death Watch*, the 1980 film adaptation of *The Continuous Katherine Mortenhoe*, Harvey Keitel plays a journalist with a camera implanted in his eye who has been assigned to befriend a dying woman, played by Romy Schneider. The film, like the book, is set in a world in which death by disease is so rare that life has lost a beauty that the frame of tragedy once provided. Keitel's character, Roddy, works for a television show, likewise called *Death Watch*, which promises viewers an immersive experience in the sweetness of untimely death.

The film's tagline: "She's the target of every eye . . . including eyes only science could create."

As in the novel, Katherine Mortenhoe is a writer who spends her days entering plot twists into a computer program that generates novels, but in the film she is not dying *of* information, instead she is dying *for* it. The producers of *Death Watch*, who have been looking for an ideally tragic star, find it in her, with her expressive face and her calm resilience. She is young enough to be beautiful, old enough to be wise, common enough to be sympathetic, extraordinary enough for TV. The producers know she is dying before she does, begin to film her in secret even as she receives the news of her fatal illness. The producers put her face on their billboards before they've even struck a deal with her for the show.

The enigmatic heroine, however, who has seen her face on that billboard and didn't like it there at all, has no interest in dying on camera. She disguises herself with a cheap wig and runs away with only a vial of prescribed painkillers in hand. She has taken the TV show's money, but not for herself, and leaves it in the hands of her mostly indifferent partner, whom she leaves, as she does everything else in her life, without notice. She sets off to die in the spare anonymity of poverty, and she suffers her pains alone in the crowd of the poor.

Roddy is the sole crew of the TV show Mortenhoe has no idea she is still starring in. With his camera eye recording, Roddy follows Mortenhoe, befriends her, and they travel to Land's End via the bleak territories of a near-future Scotland, moving among its paid protestors, housing tenements, homeless shelters, and squats. Mortenhoe wants privacy. Roddy, in his turn, needs to keep his camera eye in the light at all times—to fail to do so is to go blind. Even as he is, in one scene, in a dark jail cell, he is self-illuminated, having begged his captor for access to the light.

Mortenhoe deflects Roddy's cinematically inevitable sexual advances: this may be a movie about a man and a woman together on the road, but Mortenhoe makes emphatic that her body is too busy with dying to bother with Roddy's desire. Roddy and Mortenhoe are not lovers, but this does not mean that their relationship is not erotic. Roddy needs to see Mortenhoe and Mortenhoe needs to avoid being seen. As Mortenhoe and Roddy reach Land's End, however, Roddy has seen too much. He tosses his flashlight into the ocean, and without it, he not only loses sight, but in doing so becomes a childish wretch. Mystery, as the film makes obvious, is something that a world that loves to watch can't endure without a crisis. The light in this film is the lie: the darkness a truth the world won't allow.

Hospitals don't let the sick sleep long enough for dreams. After the last chemotherapy treatment, the drugs have damaged my body sufficiently so that I have gone from a cancer patient to a heart patient. In a cold night of January, I am alone in the critical care ward. I wake every hour among the intruders and beeps, connected to wires and tubing, freezing and worried in the hospital-white sheets.

Scholars say that in making *Hieroi Logoi*, Aelius Aristides made a public text of private remedies; a eulogy for a god inextricable from the self-celebration of a mortal; a work in which body and language twist around each other so tightly they could never be unraveled. In one of his dreams, Aristides concludes that most people's desires are the same as a pig's desires—sex, food, and sleep—but his desires are the most human because what he desires are words.

In another dream, Aristides has come across a temple built for Plato, which alarms him: we should not build temples for great people, he thinks, but instead we should write books, because while the gods are made of everything, people are the ones made out of language.

When Aristides's friends accuse him of following the prescriptions of his dreams too faithfully, he reminds them that there is no choice for him between following the directions of doctors and the directions of a god. The prescriptions Aristides follows mostly involve bathing or not bathing and a promiscuous approach to every kind of body of water. These therapeutic adventures could never be duplicated by others, as they were custom-made by the god Asclepius for only Aristides. What cures one person often kills another. The god also gave him career counseling via dreams, and following the advice of Asclepius, Aristides declaimed his speeches to the friends he had gathered around his sickbed, sometimes also writing lyric poetry for a choir of children to sing.

No route to survival is ever a clearly marked path.

In January A.D. 170, Aristides wrote that "each of our days, as well as our nights, has a story."[3] This is also true of our minutes. Half-delirious in my hospital thoughts, I attach my acquiescence to the available terminology to a large white goose and send it flying away from me into the starry night, send it away along with any petulance or vanity and my own cruelty, any personal failings that would crowd out the larger and more righteous anger.

I begin to worry that my cancer never existed, that the paranoid websites about cancer are true, that it is all a con by big pharma, that the lump was nothing, that all that had happened to me was a profitable fiction that could have been cured by carrot juice or drinking urine. In the hospital, as the cardiologists try to prove or disprove that I have a failed heart, I worry I am dying of a lie.

When Roddy goes blind, the television show *Death Watch* loses its feed. The death of Katherine Mortenhoe is no longer on the air. It is then that we learn that Katherine Mortenhoe isn't actually dying, or at least she wasn't until the TV show colluded with her doctor to give her the medicine that would create the experience of her death, pill by pill.

It is all a lie: Roddy's friendship, Mortenhoe's fatal illness, Roddy's certainty that the light will prevail, Mortenhoe's certainty that she has escaped to the darkness.

Mortenhoe is not relieved by the news that she has been tricked into believing she is dying. She is not grateful for a life extended in the same world that would kill her slowly with medicine in order that it could find pleasure in the sadness of watching her die. She takes all the deadly pills, but we are not shown her death, nor are we ever certain that she has died at all. In refusing a death scene, the film offers Mortenhoe the mystery that the world of the film tried to deny.

Two years after the filming of *Death Watch*, Romy Schneider, the actress who plays Mortenhoe, died of an overdose of pills in a Paris hotel room.

The year 1321 might be the only one in history in which the sick, infected, and disfigured organized collectively to take over their world. Or at least this was the rumor. It was believed that the lepers had planned for two years—not just for their revolt, but also the world after it. They planned who would get what and how. The wells, streams, and fountains would be simultaneously polluted with a poison—a mix of their urine and blood and four different herbs and a sanctified body. All of France (all who weren't lepers) would die or become lepers themselves. The healthy who survived the sick persons' revolt, now themselves sick people, would be the natural citizens of the sick persons' kingdom.[4]

The lepers never ruled the world: the plot was found out, the lepers were rounded up and brutalized, burned, tortured, imprisoned. Leper panic spread throughout Europe. But it is not the consequence of the lepers' plot that interests me—repression is as common as a season—it is that history contains the dream of a leper revolt at all.

"Illness," wrote the German radical group Socialist Patients' Collective, "becomes the undeniable challenge to revolutionize everything—yes, everything!—for the first time really and in the right way . . ."[5]

It's like a nurse once said to me in the infusion room: "It takes a wolf to catch a wolf."

The cardiologists have made no judgment about my heart. Because the weeks of guaranteed unpaid time off for serious illness is insufficient for anyone with serious cancer, which often inconveniences its patients by requiring that their treatment lasts a year or more and leaves them disabled at the end, I have no leave left, not for heart troubles and certainly not for all the surgeries that are still to come later in my treatment. Whether I am dying or not, I still have bills to pay, a child to support, students to teach, a job to keep: I have to go to work. I create the appearance of health from the cosmetics bag Cara brings to the hospital. The new doctor on shift in the critical care unit walks into my room where I have positioned myself as far away from the sickbed as possible. I sit upright, reading in a chair. The doctor asks me where the patient has gone.

I have been in this cancer game for months and am very tired of medicine and would prefer to say that the patient has disappeared. I instead make the medically necessary confession that I myself am the patient, and the doctor says, confounded by the contradiction between my appearance and my chart, "But you don't look sick."

This doctor, unable to reconcile my clever fabrication of health with the actuality of illness, allows me to persuade him that I can be released from the hospital despite that the conditions for which I have been admitted to the critical care unit have not changed. I am wheeled out, and because spring semester has begun, driven directly from the hospital to my workplace. I am barely able to walk the thirty steps to my classroom, can't stand, but fresh from the hospital, breathless and with a racing heart, I teach. The next morning, I go to a fourth cardiologist, who when he first sees me, says as the other one did that I do not look like the person with the heart he is reading about in the chart.

The ancient Egyptians believed that to enter the underworld, a dead person's heart—the center, to them, of the mind and of feeling—should be weighed against a feather. The heart holds an account of all of a person's deeds, if they are good or wicked, if they love or hate. Should the dead person's heart be heavier than a feather, a devourer is waiting to eat underneath the scale. Should a person's heart, however, contain the record of a life so well-lived that her heart weighs less than a feather, the person will be allowed to pass on to the afterlife.

One of the nurses from the breast surgeon's office hears that I am in the medical complex visiting the cardiologist. She tracks me down so that she can administer a hug. She is worried that I might be worried that my heart problems will prohibit the completion of my treatment—at this point, I am in the weeks between chemotherapy and mastectomy—or she herself is worried that my heart problems will prohibit the completion of my treatment, I can't tell which. I have to get the okay from cardiology before I am allowed to begin the required surgeries, and so I live strapped to a portable monitor for days, waiting for a diagnosis that the hospital cardiologists couldn't give.

It's finally resolved: my heart is not a problem. It's my nerves. The ones that regulate my heart have begun to die from the chemo, just as many of the nerves in my hands and feet have died off, too. My surgery is delayed, but not for long. I am instructed to eat food, recover, and wait for the dead parts of my body to come back to life. Mine is a heart that is hurt, but it is not a heart that is failed.

Nothing I've written here is for the well and intact, and had it been, I never would have written it. Everyone who is not sick now has been sick once or will be sick soon. I dream in elaborately missed positions, of lakes and ladders I cannot climb, of a book with the title *You Never Know and Probably Never Will*. It has as its content the worth of each life.

I know it has all been confusing, or at least it was to me, but it's the same confusion as when I am confident that every person who has ever lived knows exactly what I mean when I describe feeling like a snake on the path in the dappled sunshine that turns out, on close inspection, only to be a snake's discarded skin.

To see a snake is to also think of the way a snake slithers out of its skin, the way it has to rub its skin against something hard so that the skin begins to loosen and also the way the snake must generate sufficient new skin so that the old might be left behind. To see a snake is to think of the way the snake's eyes glaze over and it might not be able to see for a bit because there it is, getting new skin, getting rid of the old, lost in the process of becoming something else. I decide the question posed by this book is, *Are you going to be the snake or are you going to be the snake's cast-off skin?*

Just as no one is born outside of history, no one dies a natural death. Death never quits, is both universal and not. It is distributed in disproportion, arrives by drone strikes and guns and husbands' hands, is carried on the tiny backs of hospital-bred microbes, circulated in the storms raised by the new capitalist weather, arrives through a whisper of radiation instructing the mutation of a cell. It both cares who we are, and it doesn't. A squirrel has died, unmarred, of no apparent reason and is cradled at the root of a tree near my apartment. Like any mortal creature, I should not get too attached to being alive. I'd written in my journal: *In the clash of civilizations—the living versus the dead—I know whose side I'm on*, never saying which.

__ EPILOGUE

_ /and what it was that saved me

I didn't die, or at least not of this. When I got past my cancer's immediate threat, my daughter said I had done the impossible and arranged for myself to write inside a living posthumousness. After cancer, my writing felt given its full permission. I lost some neural mitochondria and my looks and many of my memories and a lot of my intelligence and an optimistically estimated five to ten years of life span to the curative forces of medical decimation, and having lost all that, found myself to still be *myself*, damaged into my own intensified version. It's like the condition of *lostness* is, when it comes to being a person, what finally makes us real.

I tried to write it all down. I spent years writing about minutes, months writing about days, weeks writing about seconds, and days writing about hours, and in the minutes of experience in which my years and days have now been lost, it still feels like the weight of these events remains too heavy for their telling. I had abandoned this book at least a thousand times, a number that does not include the innumerable other destructions inherent in writing it—the drafts deleted, pages erased, passages excised, structures disposed of, arguments unraveled, sentiments self-forbidden, anecdotes untold. This number doesn't include the Facebook account I can't stand to log back into and the tweets I've left unretrieved, or the emails I won't call up from their archive, or the hospital bills that my friends and I sailed as paper airplanes from the highest point of my city or the ones we drowned, with a plastic skeleton, in a lake. This is to say nothing, too, of the *Your Oncology Journey* binder that we buried, in pieces, after dark with kale seeds in public locations that I am not at liberty to disclose. When I hit my keyboard's space bar it was usually with a prayer that it would get stuck, that I would be allowed instead of this book an expanse of blank and cancerless pages.

If this book had to exist, I wanted it to be a minor form of reparative magic, for it to expropriate the force of literature away from literature, manifest the communism of the unlovable, grant anyone who reads it the freedom that can come from being thoroughly reduced. I wanted our lost body parts to regenerate via its sentences and for its ideas to have an elegance that will unextenuate our cells. This book could be a miracle emerging from a pile of dropped mics, announcing, as it rises, "Out of the grave and into the streets," a phrase once pronounced at a tarot reading with my friends, back when becoming a sick person was never in the works. Or if I could write the earth into opening up I would, and bring back to life an insurgent army of the dead women, but I never learned to write well enough to do all of that.

I hate to accept, but do, that cancer's near-criminal myth of singularity means any work about it always resembles testimony. It will be judged by its veracity or its utility or its depth of feeling but rarely by its form, which is its motor and its fury, which is a record of the motions of a struggle to know, if not the truth, then the weft of all competing lies.

A friend wrote about what is missing from an early draft: "There is only intermittently any Us." My response to him is, at first, *I can't lie*. But that itself is a lie, proof that I can lie and sometimes do. What I meant was that I can't pretend to have *felt* less alone, as if swimming at the lake with my friends, then having swum past them, beyond the buoys, out in the deep where no one could come to rescue me and no one I loved had ever been. And I can't account for the provenance of all that is untrue, not about cancer and not about anything else. I can't write with confidence about what has its source in species folly or my private failings or what the myopia of empire arranges to distract us from its distanced cruelty.

Oncology is a genius at the production of desolate feelings, which is why I will never believe that things were always as bad as they felt, even if they might have been worse. During diagnosis, the sick are kept in cold rooms while the technicians stand in other rooms, behind glass, talking to us through headphones. The surgeons label our body parts with purple pens. Some loved ones abandon us. Strangers fetishize our suffering. We are often so sick we can't be among others, we cease to look like ourselves, if we go among humans we are pitied as if an abandoned animal. Cancer patients, too, sometimes see in one another not comrades but cautionary tales—a tragedy we hope not to become—or someone less sick whom we must envy. Talk of shared environmental etiologies is condemned as paranoid, but the loneliness of genetic fatalism runs rampant, and so many people believe they were born with cancer's inevitability inherent in their bodies to be expunged only by surgeons or drug companies. In alternative medical environments, it's the same shit, different office park—this time with Reiki and herbs. To feel as I felt during cancer treatment is to feel like nothing at all but the saddest opportunity for profit in a world diminished so far ahead of the event of cancer that this additional diminishment is eviscerating.

But any unexamined account of desolation is a lie, or as with many truths, when submitted to the wrong context, a fraction of one. I felt desolate at the same time many others felt desolate, and before that, so many others had felt desolation ahead of me, and after me, still do. If even half of us who were sick at the same time felt the desolation of our treatment, could this vast and common loneliness be anything other than evidence that we have been fooled?

Although it is true that I often felt lonely, it is also true that my friends had moved with me in shifts through the adventure of my illness, indulging my onco-surrealist fantasies of how to be sick, allowing me to wear my thrift store silk pajamas to the movies, helping me record images of hospital vacuum cleaners and the sounds of IV drips, joining me in throwing the celebratory cake at the end of chemotherapy rather than doing as is custom and eating it. We had all agreed that if I had to have cancer, it should be experienced in a confetti storm of *amor fati*, as if performed in the mode of the 1966 anarcha-feminist film *Daisies* in which the women lie around in their underwear and set party streamers on fire. To be ruined, we said, is why the banquet exists.

My friend Cara told me that it was clear that when I was at my lowest, what I needed most was art—not comfort—and so it was to get through cancer that I had to wish everything around me into aesthetic extremity. I had needed to daydream of coffins filled with embalming honey, invent speculative religions, write polemics, take revenge, and conceive of a brand-new version of the funerary, making lists of all the miniature electronics our souls should take with us to the afterworld, which I also tried to reinvent.

During my treatment, some of my friends sent me cannabis popcorn wrapped in the poet Diane di Prima's hand-me-down yoga pants. I had no partner to take care of me, but their gift was proof that I had the better part of the world, and despite every argument for inescapability made by the world's structures of deprivation, deprivation is not the entire world. Cancer was hard, but I had these inventive forms of love to soften it, even if these loves were the completely extralegal and unofficial kind, unattached to the couple or family. But when I was sick, I also felt the cold sadness of what would have happened if I was friendless or for whatever reason at that point unlovable, or what might happen to me when I became so. Some friends left, but some friends patchworked their money and time into care for me. The ones who had money wrote checks so that the ones with the capacity for thoughtful care could fly to me and help me empty the surgical drains stitched into my body. Some friends sent books, others sent mixtapes. Our solution to the problem of care is not scalable, was inadequate and provisional, but at least it got me through.

Once during treatment when the tumor hurt and felt like it was growing again and I was terrified of a painful and lonely death, my friend Jasper sat on the sofa I'd moved to the dining room so that whoever came to visit to take care of me would have a place to sleep. Jasper seemed uninterested in the practice of turning on and off lights, and I had convinced myself that as a woman, I would be acting out of internalized oppression if I compensated for this by turning on and off the lights for us. That's how we ended up discussing merciful death on this sofa in an almost completely dark room full of functional lamps. Jasper answered my fear of the painful and humiliating death by this cancer with "Well, we'll all just make sure that doesn't happen." I believed him of course, that despite the risks my friends would help me die according to my own desires, because my friends had been so mostly reliable and generous and resourceful during my illness. Yet at the thought of leaving my friends behind forever I began to cry and fled to my room.

I'd hoped he hadn't noticed I was crying: these were silent tears and everything was dark and sometimes he gave an air of being too smart to notice what was happening on another person's face. But I was in my room for only a minute when I saw that he had followed me. I then said, in that high tight voice of totally unconvincing protest, "I'm okay!" but wasn't, and he suggested that this would be a good time to watch some TV.

So we did, and in the dim flicker of a *Black Mirror* episode in the living room, I thought about all the women writers who had died early and who I wished had lived. Mary Wollstonecraft was thirty-eight when she died after giving birth to Mary Shelley. The nineteenth-century French-Peruvian socialist philosopher Flora Tristan was forty-one when she died of exhaustion after trying to organize France's working class. The philosopher Margaret Fuller was forty when she died, drowning off the coast of Fire Island, "her hair loose over her white dress, facing America," her last words: "I see nothing but death before me."[1]

Before I got sick, the work of these dead women had kept me company. They had imagined a new structure to the world and with it, the world's real possibilities. And in my forty-first year I gathered these writers around me, too, detached myself from the things of the living little by little. I imagined a new structure for the world, as I always did, then rehearsed my death, peeled desire away from me as if taking off clothes. My activity narrowed, my attachments narrowed: then my ambitions abstracted—I was able to love from a length and through this, to imagine love's larger form.

Mortality is a gorgeous framework. What a relief to have not been protected, I decided, to not be a subtle or delicate person whose inner experience is made only of taste and polite feeling; what a relief not to collect tiny wounds as if they are the greatest injuries while all the rest of the world always, really, actually bleeds. It's yet another error in perception that those with social protection can look at those who have at times lacked it, and imagine that weakness is in the bleeder, not those who have never bled. Those who diminish the beauty and luxury of survival must do so because they have been so rarely almost dead.

I'd survived, yet the ideological regime of cancer means that to call myself a *survivor* still feels like a betrayal of the dead. But I'll admit that not a day passes in which I am not ecstatic that I still get to live. I am sorry that I was not able to write down everything. The great orbs of the unsaid continue to float through the air. *But it is time for a new problem*, the horizontal has said to the vertical. Then the moon, once so obsessed with waning, finally waxed.

NOTES

PROLOGUE

1. Susan Sontag and David Rieff. *As Consciousness Is Harnessed to Flesh: Journals and Notebooks, 1964–1980.* New York: Picador, 2013.
2. Alice James and Leon Edel. *The Diary of Alice James.* Boston: Northeastern University Press, 1999.
3. Susan Sontag. *Illness As Metaphor.* New York: Farrar, Straus and Giroux, 1978.
4. Ellen Leopold. *A Darker Ribbon: Breast Cancer, Women, and Their Doctors in the Twentieth Century.* Boston: Beacon Press, 2000.
5. Sontag, *As Consciousness Is Harnessed to Flesh.*
6. Jacqueline Susann. *Valley of the Dolls: A Novel.* New York: Bantam Books, 1966.
7. Charlotte Perkins Gilman. *The Living of Charlotte Perkins Gilman: An Autobiography.* Salem, N.H.: Ayer, 1987.
8. Audre Lorde. *The Cancer Journals.* San Francisco: Aunt Lute Books, 2006.
9. Fanny Burney, Barbara G. Schrank, and David J. Supino. *The Famous Miss Burney: The Diaries and Letters of Fanny Burney.* New York: John Day, 1976.
10. Sontag, *As Consciousness Is Harnessed to Flesh.*
11. Kathy Acker. "The Gift of Disease." *The Guardian*, January 18, 1997, p. T14.
12. Lorde, *The Cancer Journals.*
13. Sontag, *As Consciousness Is Harnessed to Flesh.*
14. Eve Kosofsky Sedgwick. *A Dialogue on Love.* Boston: Beacon Press, 2006.
15. S. Lochlann Jain. *Malignant: How Cancer Becomes Us.* Berkeley: University of California Press, 2013.
16. Ibid.
17. Leopold, *A Darker Ribbon.*
18. Lorde, *The Cancer Journals.*
19. Sontag, *As Consciousness Is Harnessed to Flesh.*

THE INCUBANTS

1. BI-RADS (Breast Imaging-Reporting and Data System) is a quality control system for reading mammograms, trademarked by the American College of Radiology (ACR). A score of 5 on the BI-RADS scale indicates more than a 95 percent chance of malignancy.

2. Aelius Aristides and Charles A. Behr. *Aelius Aristides and the Sacred Tales.* Amsterdam: Hakkert, 1969.

3. Lee T. Pearcy. "Theme, Dream, and Narrative: Reading the Sacred Tales of Aelius Aristides." *Transactions of the American Philological Association (1974–)*, vol. 118, 1988.

4. Michael T. Compton. "The Union of Religion and Health in Ancient Asklepieia." *Journal of Religion and Health*, vol. 37, no. 4, 1998.

5. Created by the Cancer Math group at the Laboratory for Quantitative Medicine at Massachusetts General Hospital, LifeMath's breast cancer contributions include Conditional Survival, Nipple Involvement, Nodal Status, Therapy, and Outcomes calculators. The outcomes of cancer when these variables are entered into the calculators is demonstrated via mortality curves, survival curves, pictograms, bar graphs, and pie charts, a set of choices offered in a drop-down menu.

6. Metastatic breast cancer, fake boobs, and No Evidence of Disease, respectively.

7. According to the Wage and Hour Division of the U.S. Department of Labor, the twelve-week Family and Medical Leave Act that covers full-time U.S. workers only guarantees (unpaid) time off to care for "the employee's spouse, child, or parent who has a serious health condition."

8. Siddhartha Mukherjee. *The Emperor of All Maladies.* London: HarperCollins, 2017.

9. Ki-67 is a nuclear protein associated with cellular proliferation, and its overexpression has been correlated with poorer survival outcomes in cancer patients.

10. Neoadjuvant chemotherapy, which means chemotherapy before surgery, is not common in breast cancer treatment, except in cases of aggressive cancers or large tumors. An advantage of neoadjuvant chemotherapy for people with triple-negative breast cancer is that it allows monitoring of the tumor site for a "pathologic complete response," which means that all signs of cancer have been wiped out by chemotherapy.

11. Mukherjee, *The Emperor of All Maladies.*

12. Carlo Ginzburg's essay "Clues: Roots of an Evidential Paradigm," in *Clues, Myths, and the Historical Method* (see bibliography), had a

significant influence over my thinking about what effect the diagnostic process can have on lived experience. Ginzburg describes the Morellian method, developed by the nineteenth-century art historian Giovanni Morelli, which involves determining the authenticity of a painting through careful study of minor details such as earlobes and fingernails. Ginzburg links the Morellian method with the approaches of Sherlock Holmes and Sigmund Freud. In all of these methods, and in cancer diagnosis, too, what appears to be unimportant becomes the most closely examined thing. As a result, what once was only itself soon becomes "evidence," and in the case of cancer diagnosis and criminal investigation, the kind that can damn a person for life.

13. John Cage. *A Year from Monday: New Lectures and Writings*. Middletown, Conn.: Wesleyan University Press, 1969.
14. I use the term "ideology" in this book to mean a version of shared reality that arises from historical circumstances. Ideology often *feels* so natural or so true to us that it remains unexamined in daily life, assumed to be the actual truth until we confront a painful demonstration of its falsehood. In my experience, a crisis like breast cancer tends to promote the overproduction of the ideological and, through this, generates so many contradictions and dissonances that eventually what is generally accepted but untrue becomes rapidly exposed, with no other truth—at least not the shared kind—to immediately take its place.
15. John Donne and Izaak Walton. *Devotions upon Emergent Occasions: And, Death's Duel*. New York: Vintage Books, 1999.
16. Ibid.
17. Clarice Lispector, Stefan Tobler, and Benjamin Moser. *Agua Viva*. London: Penguin Classics, 2014.
18. Aristides, *Sacred Tales*.

BIRTH OF THE PAVILION

1. Donne, *Devotions upon Emergent Occasions*.
2. Fran Lowry. "'Chemo Brain': MRI Shows Brain Changes After Chemotherapy." *Medscape*, Nov. 16, 2011, www.medscape.com/viewarticle/753663.
3. Tim Newman. "How Long Does 'Chemo Brain' Last?" Medical News Today, *MediLexicon International*, Aug. 19, 2016, www.medicalnewstoday.com/articles/312436.php.
4. Michel Foucault. *The Birth of the Clinic*, 3rd ed. London: Routledge, 2017.

5. G. Cassinelli. "The Roots of Modern Oncology: From Discovery of New Antitumor Anthracyclines to Their Clinical Use." *Advances in Pediatrics*, U.S. National Library of Medicine, June 2, 2016, www.ncbi.nlm.nih.gov/pubmed/27103205.

6. Sarah Hazell. "Mustard Gas—from the Great War to Frontline Chemotherapy." *Cancer Research UK—Science Blog*, Aug. 24, 2014, scienceblog.cancerresearchuk.org/2014/08/27/mustard-gas-from-the-great-war-to-frontline-chemotherapy/.

7. From the back of a jean jacket worn by the artist/activist David Wojnarowicz in 1988: "If I die of AIDS—forget burial—just drop my body on the steps of the F.D.A."

8. According to the American Cancer Society website, "The Look Good Feel Better program was founded and developed in 1989 by the Personal Care Products Council (at the time called the Cosmetic, Toiletry and Fragrance Association, or CTFA), a charitable organization supported by the cosmetic industry, in cooperation with the American Cancer Society (ACS) and the Professional Beauty Association (or PBA), a national organization that represents hairstylists, wig experts, estheticians, makeup artists, and other professionals in the cosmetic industry." This two-hour workshop for women with cancer distributes free makeup kits along with advice on how to camouflage "areas of concern." According to Breast Cancer Action, "Many of these donated products contain chemicals linked to increasing cancer risk and can actually interfere with breast cancer treatment."

9. While not yet as ubiquitous as pink ribbon products, there are currently enough varieties of "Fuck Cancer" T-shirts that a person could dress exclusively in "Fuck Cancer" T-shirts for at least a month, and probably two, and never have to repeat a shirt or do laundry. It has also become a popular slogan to engrave into jewelry, including one product from Etsy that combines "Fuck Cancer" with "This too shall pass."

10. Ester Heath et al. "Fate and Effects of the Residues of Anticancer Drugs in the Environment." *SpringerLink*, June 28, 2016, link.springer.com/article/10.1007/s11356-016-7069-3.

11. Hanna Gersmann and Jessica Aldred. "Medicinal Tree Used in Chemotherapy Drug Faces Extinction." *The Guardian*, Nov. 10, 2011, www.theguardian.com/environment/2011/nov/10/iucn-red-list-tree-chemotherapy.

12. Meg Tirrell. "The World Spent This Much on Cancer Drugs Last Year . . ." CNBC, June 2, 2016, www.cnbc.com/2016/06/02/the-worlds-2015-cancer-drug-bill-107-billion-dollars.html.

THE SICKBED

1. John Donne and Herbert J. C. Grierson. *The Poems of John Donne.* Oxford, U.K.: Oxford University Press, 2011.
2. Harriet Martineau. *Life in the Sick-Room: Essays, by an Invalid*, 3rd ed. London: Edward Moxon, 1849. The invalid was Martineau herself.
3. Virginia Woolf, Julia D. Stephen, Hermione Lee, Mark Hussey, and Rita Charon. *On Being Ill.* Ashfield, Mass.: Paris Press, 2012.
4. Donne, *Devotions upon Emergent Occasions.*
5. Woolf et al., *On Being Ill.*
6. Nicole Loraux. *Tragic Ways of Killing a Woman.* Cambridge, Mass.: Harvard University Press, 1992.
7. Plutarchus and Christopher B. R. Pelling. *Life of Antony.* Cambridge, U.K.: Cambridge University Press, 2005.
8. Marlene Dumas and Mariska Berg. *Sweet Nothings: Notes and Texts, 1982–2014.* London: Tate Publishing, 2015.
9. Woolf et al., *On Being Ill.*
10. Leviticus 13:45: "And the leper in whom the plague is, his clothes shall be rent, and his head bare, and he shall put a covering upon his upper lip, and shall cry, Unclean, unclean."
11. Diane di Prima. *Revolutionary Letters.* San Francisco: City Lights Books, 1974.
12. Johann W. Goethe and Charles T. Brooks. *Faust: A Tragedy.* Boston: Houghton, Osgood and Co., 1880.
13. Later in the same scene, Faust says this to his poodle companion:

    > We know that men will treat with derision
    > Whatever they cannot understand.

14. Bertolt Brecht, Tom Kuhn, Steve Giles, and Laura J. R. Bradley. *Brecht on Art and Politics.* London: Methuen, 2003.
15. Ibid.
16. Aristides, *Sacred Tales.*

HOW THE ORACLE HELD

1. Avicenna: "We say: If a human is created all at once, created with his limbs separated and he does not see them, and if it happens that he does not touch them and they do not touch each other, and he hears

no sound, he would be ignorant of the existence of the whole of his organs, but would know the existence of his individual being as one thing, while being ignorant of all the former things. What is itself the unknown is not the known."

2. Lucretius, from Book III of *De rerum natura*:

> We often see
> Men die by inches; toes and nails succumb
> To lividness, next feet and legs, till soon
> The other limbs feel the chill tread of death.
> And since the same thing happens to the spirit,
> Which never seems to issue, all at once,
> Out of the body, it is also mortal.

3. D. G. Compton and Jeff VanderMeer. *The Continuous Katherine Mortenhoe*. New York: New York Review Books, 2016.
4. Ibid.
5. Ibid.
6. Ibid.
7. Burney, *Diaries and Letters*.
8. Lorde, *The Cancer Journals*.
9. Despite the historical differences in the circumstances around our mastectomies, Lorde also had to wake up from her surgery fighting, but in Lorde's case, it was for the basic right to make noise when in pain. As she writes in *The Cancer Journals*, "I remember screaming and cursing with pain in the recovery room, and I remember a disgusted nurse giving me a shot. I remember a voice telling me to be quiet because there were sick people here, and my saying, well, I have a right, because I'm sick, too."
10. Julie Appleby. "More Women Are Having Mastectomies and Going Home the Same Day." NPR, Feb. 22, 2016, www.npr.org/sections /health-shots/2016/02/22/467644987/more-women-are-having -mastectomies-and-going-home-that-day.

THE HOAX

1. Ray Leszcynski. "'He Had Us All Duped': Mesquite Teacher's Aide Has Criminal Past, Not Cancer." *Dallas Morning News*, Jan. 24, 2017, www.dallasnews.com/news/crime/2017/01/24/us-duped-mesquite -teachers-aide-federal-court-sentencing-date-cancer.
2. Hannah Button. "Friends Question Tualatin Woman's Cancer Diag-

nosis." KOIN, June 20, 2017, www.koin.com/news/friends-question
-tualatin-womans-cancer-diagnosis_20171130084913371
/870074736.

3. Crystal Bui. "Woonsocket Woman Accused of Faking Cancer,
Spending Donations." WJAR News, June 22, 2017, turnto10.com/news
/local/woonsocket-woman-accused-of-faking-cancer-to-raise
-money.

4. "Society Can Decide If 15-Year Term Is Enough for Jailed Surgeon,
Victim Says." *Herald Scotland*, May 31, 2017, www.heraldscotland
.com/news/15319719.Society_can_decide_if_15_year_term_is
_enough_for_jailed_surgeon__victim_says/.

5. "Belle Gibson | The Whole Pantry." *ELLE*, Mar. 13, 2015, www.elle
.com.au/news/what-we-know-about-belle-gibson-5919.

6. Robert Allen. "Cancer Doctor Sentenced to 45 Years for 'Horrific'
Fraud." *USA Today*, Gannett Satellite Information Network,
July 11, 2015, www.usatoday.com/story/news/nation/2015/07/10
/cancer-doctor-sentenced-years-horrific-fraud/29996107/.

7. Martin Fricker. "Breast Surgeon Who 'Played God with Women'
Faces More Jail Time." *Coventry Telegraph*, Dec. 27, 2017, www
.coventrytelegraph.net/news/local-news/demon-breast-surgeon
-who-played-13350152.

8. Alice Park. "Great Science Frauds." *TIME*, Jan. 12, 2012, healthland
.time.com/2012/01/13/great-science-frauds/slide/dr-roger-poisson/.

9. "FDA Warning Letter to Sanofi-Aventis Re Taxotere Marketing."
FierceBiotech, May 14, 2009, www.fiercebiotech.com/biotech/fda
-warning-letter-to-sanofi-aventis-re-taxotere-marketing.

10. Katie Thomas. "Celgene to Pay $280 Million to Settle Fraud Suit
over Cancer Drugs." *The New York Times*, July 26, 2017, www
.nytimes.com/2017/07/25/health/celgene-to-pay-280-million-to
-settle-fraud-suit-over-cancer-drugs.html.

11. "Consumer Updates—Products Claiming To." *U.S. Food and Drug
Administration Home Page*, Center for Biologics Evaluation and Research, www.fda.gov/forconsumers/consumerupdates/ucm048383
.htm.

12. "Gainsborough Woman Whose Elaborate Cancer Hoax Conned
Employer out of £14,000 Is Ordered to Pay Back £1." *Gainsborough
Standard* (U.K.), June 19, 2017, www.gainsboroughstandard.co.uk
/news/gainsborough-woman-whose-elaborate-cancer-hoax
-conned-employer-out-of-14-000-is-ordered-to-pay-back-1-1
-8604627.

13. Caitlin C. "In Memoriam: Charlotte Haley, Creator of the First
(Peach) Breast Cancer Ribbon." *Breast Cancer Action*, June 24, 2014,

www.bcaction.org/2014/06/24/in-memoriam-charlotte-haley
-creator-of-the-first-peach-breast-cancer-ribbon/.

14. "History of the Pink Ribbon." *Think Before You Pink*, thinkbefore
-youpink.org/resources/history-of-the-pink-ribbon/.

15. Susan G. Komen for the Cure. "The Pink Ribbon Story." https://ww5
.komen.org/uploadedfiles/content_binaries/the_pink_ribbon
_story.pdf.

16. "Komen to Reformulate Perfume after Unfavorable Allegations."
www.nbcdfw.com/news/local/Komen-to-Reformulate-Perfume
-After-Unfavorable-Allegations-131338323.html.

17. Caitlin C. "Susan G. Komen Partners with Global Fracking Corporation to Launch 'Benzene and Formaldehyde for the Cure°.'" *Breast
Cancer Action*, Dec. 2, 2014, www.bcaction.org/2014/10/08/susan-g
-komen-partners-with-global-fracking-corporation-to-launch
-benzene-and-formaldehyde-for-the-cure/.

18. Erik Eckholm. "$89 Million Awarded Family Who Sued H.M.O."
The New York Times, Dec. 30, 1993, www.nytimes.com/1993/12/30
/us/89-million-awarded-family-who-sued-hmo.html.

19. Richard A. Rettig. *False Hope: Bone Marrow Transplantation for
Breast Cancer*. Oxford, U.K.: Oxford University Press, 2007.

20. Denise Grady. "Breast Cancer Researcher Admits Falsifying Data."
The New York Times, Feb. 5, 2000, www.nytimes.com/2000/02/05/us
/breast-cancer-researcher-admits-falsifying-data.html.

21. "Majority of Women Diagnosed with Breast Cancer after Screening
Mammograms Get Unnecessary Treatment, Study Finds." *Los Angeles Times*, Oct. 12, 2016, www.latimes.com/science/sciencenow/la
-sci-sn-breast-cancer-screening-mammograms-20161012-snap
-story.html.

22. Christie Aschwanden et al. "What If Everything Your Doctors Told
You About Breast Cancer Was Wrong?" *Mother Jones*, June 24, 2017,
www.motherjones.com/politics/2015/10/faulty-research-behind
-mammograms-breast-cancer/.

23. Acker, "The Gift of Disease."

24. Sarah Schulman. *Gentrification of the Mind: Witness to a Lost
Imagination*. Berkeley: University of California Press, 2013.

25. "The Last Days of Kathy Acker." *Hazlitt*, July 30, 2015, hazlitt.net
/feature/last-days-kathy-acker.

26. Lauren Elkin. "*After Kathy Acker* by Chris Kraus—Radical Empa-
thy." *Financial Times*, Aug. 11, 2017, www.ft.com/content/b4ce8f48
-7dc5-11e7-ab01-a13271d1ee9c.

27. Acker, "The Gift of Disease."

28. Ibid.

29. Chris Kraus. *After Kathy Acker: A Biography*. London: Penguin Books, 2018.
30. Audre Lorde and Rudolph P. Byrd. *I Am Your Sister: Collected and Unpublished Writings of Audre Lorde*. Singapore: Oxford University Press, 2011.

IN THE TEMPLE OF GIULIETTA MASINA'S TEARS

1. Elaine Scarry. *The Body in Pain: The Making and Unmaking of the World*. New York: Oxford University Press, 1985.
2. Roselyne Rey. *The History of Pain*. Cambridge, Mass.: Harvard University Press, 1998.
3. The Wound Man is an anatomical drawing used to illustrate common accidents and injuries, and first appeared in medical texts in 1491. This illustration of the Wound Man is from Hans von Gersdorff's *Feldtbuch der Wundartzney* (Fieldbook of Surgery), 1519. Despite the Wound Man's multiple injuries, he is always depicted upright and alive.
4. This cadaver skin comes from organ and tissue donors, many of whom do not know that their tissue will be immediately harvested and trafficked through a chain of for-profit corporations. LifeCell promises that cadaver skin for bilateral breast reconstruction will be sourced from the same donor—so although I have two pieces of cadaver skin in me, it is only from a single person—but Alloderm is used not only to help cancer patients and other sick people, but can be used, as well, for elective cosmetic surgeries unrelated to illness. Although the for-profit tissue world remains murky, a 2017 investigative series by Reuters called "The Body Trade" points out that it is generally not illegal in the United States to sell human cadavers. Industry estimates are that donated tissue sales bring in millions of dollars in profits each year, none of this going to the loved ones of the donors: www.reuters.com/investigates/section/usa-bodies/.
5. An illustration of the pathway of pain from the philosopher René Descartes's *Treatise on Man*, 1664.

DEATHWATCH

1. Aristides, *Sacred Tales*.
2. Cathérine Peyroux. "The Leper's Kiss." In *Monks & Nuns, Saints & Outcasts: Religion in Medieval Society: Essays in Honor of Lester K.*

Little, edited by Sharon Farmer and Barbara H. Rosenwein. Ithaca, N.Y.: Cornell University Press, 2000.

3. Aristides, *Sacred Tales*.
4. Carlo Ginzburg. *Ecstasies: Deciphering the Witches' Sabbath*. Chicago: University of Chicago Press, 2004.
5. SPK (Socialist Patients' Collective). *Turn Illness into a Weapon: For Agitation*. Heidelberg: KRRIM, 1993.

EPILOGUE

1. John Matteson. *The Lives of Margaret Fuller: A Biography*. New York: W. W. Norton, 2013.

BIBLIOGRAPHY

Acker, Kathy. "The Gift of Disease." *The Guardian*, January 18, 1997, p. T14.

Arendt, Hannah, et al. *The Human Condition*. Chicago: University of Chicago Press, 2018.

Aristides, Aelius, and Charles A. Behr. *Aelius Aristides and the Sacred Tales*. Amsterdam: Hakkert, 1969.

Avicenna, and Shams C. Inati. *Ibn Sina's Remarks and Admonitions: Physics and Metaphysics: An Analysis and Annotated Translation*. New York: Columbia University Press, 2014.

Bellamy, Dodie. *When the Sick Rule the World*. South Pasadena, Calif.: Semiotext(e), 2015.

Berkowitz, Amy. *Tender Points*. Oakland, Calif.: Timeless Infinite Light, 2015.

Biss, Eula. "The Pain Scale." *Harper's Magazine*, 2005.

Brecht, Bertolt, Tom Kuhn, Steve Giles, and Laura J. R. Bradley. *Brecht on Art and Politics*. London: Methuen, 2003.

Burney, Fanny, Barbara G. Schrank, and David J. Supino. *The Famous Miss Burney: The Diaries and Letters of Fanny Burney*. New York: John Day, 1976.

Burnham, John C. *What Is Medical History?* Cambridge, U.K.: Polity, 2007.

Cage, John. *A Year from Monday: New Lectures and Writings*. Middletown, Conn.: Wesleyan University Press, 1969.

Cazdyn, Eric M. *The Already Dead: The New Time of Politics, Culture, and Illness*. Durham: Duke University Press, 2012.

Compton, D. G., and Jeff VanderMeer. *The Continuous Katherine Mortenhoe*. New York: New York Review Books, 2016.

Compton, Michael T. "The Union of Religion and Health in Ancient Asklepieia." *Journal of Religion and Health*, vol. 37, no. 4, 1998.

Di Prima, Diane. *Revolutionary Letters*. San Francisco: City Lights Books, 1974.

Donne, John, and Herbert J. C. Grierson. *The Poems of John Donne*. Oxford, U.K.: Oxford University Press, 2011.

Donne, John, and Izaak Walton. *Devotions upon Emergent Occasions: And, Death's Duel.* New York: Vintage Books, 1999.

Dumas, Marlene, and Mariska Berg. *Sweet Nothings: Notes and Texts, 1982–2014.* London: Tate Publishing, 2015.

Fenton, James, Alphonse Daudet, and Julian Barnes. "In the Land of Pain." *The New York Review of Books*, vol. 50, no. 2, 2003.

Foucault, Michel. *The Birth of the Clinic*, 3rd. ed. London: Routledge, 2017.

Gilman, Charlotte Perkins. *The Living of Charlotte Perkins Gilman: An Autobiography.* Salem, N.H.: Ayer, 1987.

Ginzburg, Carlo. *Ecstasies: Deciphering the Witches' Sabbath.* Chicago: University of Chicago Press, 2004.

Ginzburg, Carlo, John Tedeschi, and Anne C. Tedeschi. *Clues, Myths, and the Historical Method.* Baltimore: Johns Hopkins University Press, 2013.

Goethe, Johann W., and Charles T. Brooks. *Faust: A Tragedy.* Boston: Houghton, Osgood and Co., 1880.

Israelowich, Ido. *Society, Medicine and Religion in the Sacred Tales of Aelius Aristides.* Leiden: Brill, 2012.

Jain, S. Lochlann. *Malignant: How Cancer Becomes Us.* Berkeley: University of California Press, 2013.

James, Alice, and Leon Edel. *The Diary of Alice James.* Boston: Northeastern University Press, 1999.

King, Samantha. *Pink Ribbons, Inc: Breast Cancer and the Politics of Philanthropy.* Minneapolis: University of Minnesota Press, 2008.

Kraus, Chris. *After Kathy Acker: A Biography.* London: Penguin Books, 2018.

Leopold, Ellen. *A Darker Ribbon: Breast Cancer, Women, and Their Doctors in the Twentieth Century.* Boston: Beacon Press, 2000.

Levinas, Emmanuel, and Seán Hand. *The Levinas Reader.* Malden, Mass.: Blackwell, 2009.

Lispector, Clarice, Stefan Tobler, and Benjamin Moser. *Agua Viva.* London: Penguin Classics, 2014.

Loraux, Nicole. *Tragic Ways of Killing a Woman.* Cambridge, Mass.: Harvard University Press, 1992.

Lord, Catherine. *The Summer of Her Baldness: A Cancer Improvisation.* Austin: University of Texas Press, 2004.

Lorde, Audre. *The Audre Lorde Compendium: Essays, Speeches, and Journals.* London: Pandora, 1996.

———. *The Cancer Journals.* San Francisco: Aunt Lute Books, 2006.

Lorde, Audre, and Rudolph P. Byrd. *I Am Your Sister: Collected and Un-*

published Writings of Audre Lorde. Singapore: Oxford University Press, 2011.

Lucretius and Rolfe Humphries. *The Way Things Are: The "De Rerum Natura" of Titus Lucretius Carus.* Bloomington: Indiana University Press, 1968.

Martineau, Harriet. *Life in the Sick-Room: Essays, by an Invalid.* 3rd ed. London: Edward Moxon, 1849.

Matteson, John. *The Lives of Margaret Fuller: A Biography.* New York: W. W. Norton, 2013.

Mukherjee, Siddhartha. *The Emperor of All Maladies.* London: Harper-Collins, 2017.

Pearcy, Lee T. "Theme, Dream, and Narrative: Reading the Sacred Tales of Aelius Aristides." *Transactions of the American Philological Association (1974–),* vol. 118, 1988.

Petsalēs-Diomēdēs, Alexia. *"Truly Beyond Wonders": Aelius Aristides and the Cult of Asklepios.* Oxford, U.K.: Oxford University Press, 2010.

Peyroux, Cathérine. "The Leper's Kiss." In *Monks & Nuns, Saints & Outcasts: Religion in Medieval Society: Essays in Honor of Lester K. Little,* edited by Sharon Farmer and Barbara H. Rosenwein. Ithaca, N.Y.: Cornell University Press, 2000.

Plutarchus and Christopher B. R. Pelling. *Life of Antony.* Cambridge, U.K.: Cambridge University Press, 2005.

Rettig, Richard A. *False Hope: Bone Marrow Transplantation for Breast Cancer.* Oxford, U.K.: Oxford University Press, 2007.

Rey, Roselyne. *The History of Pain.* Cambridge, Mass.: Harvard University Press, 1998.

Rousseau, Jean-Jacques, et al. *The First and Second Discourses Together with the Replies to Critics; and, Essay on the Origin of Languages.* New York: Harper & Row, 1986.

Scarry, Elaine. *The Body in Pain: The Making and Unmaking of the World.* New York: Oxford University Press, 1985.

Schulman, Sarah. *Gentrification of the Mind: Witness to a Lost Imagination.* Berkeley: University of California Press, 2013.

Sedgwick, Eve Kosofsky. *A Dialogue on Love.* Boston: Beacon Press, 2006.

Sontag, Susan. *Illness As Metaphor.* New York: Farrar, Straus and Giroux, 1978.

Sontag, Susan, and David Rieff. *As Consciousness Is Harnessed to Flesh: Journals and Notebooks, 1964–1980.* New York: Picador, 2013.

SPK (Socialist Patients' Collective). *Turn Illness into a Weapon: For Agitation.* Heidelberg: KRRIM, 1993.

Stephens, John. *The Dreams and Visions of Aelius Aristides: A Case-Study in the History of Religions.* Piscataway, N.J.: Gorgias Press, 2013.

Susann, Jacqueline. *Valley of the Dolls: A Novel.* New York: Bantam Books, 1966.

Woolf, Virginia, Julia D. Stephen, Hermione Lee, Mark Hussey, and Rita Charon. *On Being Ill.* Ashfield, Mass.: Paris Press, 2012.

ACKNOWLEDGMENTS

Thank you to all the people whose care, conversation, encouragement, feedback, and example helped make this book possible, particularly CAConrad, Louis-Georges Schwartz, Jonathan Kissam, Erin Morril, Juliana Spahr, Dana Ward, Jasper Bernes, Daniel Spaulding, Sandra Simonds, Magdalena Zurawski, David Buuck, Anthony Iles, Jenny Diski, Ariana Reines, Carolyn Lazard, Dan Hoy, Amalle Dublon, Emma Heaney, Evan Calder-Williams, Jonah Criswell, Cyrus Console-Soicon, Jordan Stempleman, Phyllis Moore, Jonathan Lethem, Josh Honn, Frank Sherlock, Lauren Levin, Aaron Kunin, Hari Kunzru, Natalia Cecire, Jace Clayton, Lisa Robertson, Lyn Hejinian, Joanna Hedva, Sampson Starkweather, Constantina Zavitsanos, Malcolm Harris, Ed Luker, Jacob Bard-Rosenberg, Melissa Flashman, and Jeremy M. Davies. L. E. Long, Cara Lefebvre, Cassandra Gillig, and Hazel Carson deserve special thanks. Most of what is good in this book is because of them. I also want to thank all the workers who helped take care of me during my illness, the technicians, nurses, paraprofessionals, doctors, clerical workers, cleaners, EMIs, and others who kept me safe and calm through this harrowing experience.

Some of this writing has appeared in *The New Inquiry*, the Poetry Foundation's *Harriet* blog, *Litmus*, *Swimmers*, and *Guernica*. "Wasted Life" was part of a project commissioned by EMPAC for an exhibit by Patricia Lennox-Boyd. Some of the writing and thinking about care came from a talk given at the British Columbia Nurses' Union conference in 2015, and some of the writing about Kathy Acker came from a talk given at an event at the CUNY grad center about Chris Kraus's *After Kathy Acker*. I want to thank these editors and event organizers who helped bring this work into the world.

So much of my thinking, too, has emerged from conversations on social media, over email, and after readings and events, and I want to thank all of the generous interlocutors—many of whom have shared similar experiences with illness and disability—who have given me the ongoing opportunity to understand the world. I also want to acknowledge the thousands of people who make up the online communities that have gathered around breast cancer. Their emails, Facebook posts, tweets, vlogs, and forum contributions—all offered freely and in the interest of helping others—were necessary to my understanding of my experience. In particular, those who shared their lives on video, like Coopdizzle and Christina Newman, made a profound impact on me both during and after my treatment.

This work has been made possible with faculty development funds from the Kansas City Art Institute and a Philip Whalen Grant from Poets in Need. I also want to thank the Whiting Foundation, the Foundation for Contemporary Arts, and the Judith E. Wilson fund at Cambridge University for recognizing my work and providing me with the material support necessary for the completion of this book.

A Note About the Author

Anne Boyer is a poet and an essayist who lives in Kansas City. Her honors include the 2018 Cy Twombly Award for Poetry from the Foundation for Contemporary Art, a 2018 Whiting Award in nonfiction/poetry, and the 2018–2019 Judith E. Wilson Fellowship in poetry at Cambridge University. She is the author of several collections of poetry, including the 2016 CLMP Firecracker Award–winning *Garments Against Women*, and a book of fables, essays, and ephemera titled *A Handbook of Disappointed Fate*.